HEALTH MANPOWER PLANNING

Health Manpower Planning

Methods and Strategies for the Maintenance of Standards and for Cost-Control

Proceedings of a European Symposium held at the University of Limburg, Maastricht, The Netherlands, April 14-16, 1982

edited by

FRANS C.A. JASPERS, M.D.
ALVIN R. TARLOV, M.D.
ERIC L. VRIJLAND, M.D.

1983 **MARTINUS NIJHOFF PUBLISHERS**
a member of the KLUWER ACADEMIC PUBLISHERS GROUP
BOSTON / THE HAGUE / DORDRECHT / LANCASTER
for the Permanent Working Group of European Junior Hospital Doctors

The Symposium was organized by the DUTCH and SWEDISH ASSOCIATIONS OF JUNIOR HOSPITAL DOCTORS (LVAG and SYLF), and the FACULTY OF MEDICINE OF THE UNIVERSIT OF LIMBURG, Maastricht, The Netherlands.
The PERMANENT WORKING GROUP OF EUROPEAN JUNIOR HOSPITAL DOCTORS (PWG) had the auspices.

Distributors

for the United States and Canada: Kluwer Boston, Inc., 190 Old Derby Street, Hingham, MA 02043, USA
for all other countries: Kluwer Academic Publishers Group, Distribution Center,P.O.Box 322, 3300 AH Dordrecht, The Netherlands

Library of Congress Cataloging in Publication Data

Main entry under title:

Health manpower planning.

"Proceedings of a European Symposium held in the University Limburg at Maastricht, the Netherlands, April 14-16, 1982 ... organized by the Dutch and Swedish associations of junior hospital doctors (LVAG and SYIF), and the Faculty of Medicine of the University Limburg at Maastricht, the Netherlands."
1. Medical personnel--European Economic Community countries--Congresses. 2. Health planning--European Economic Community countries--Congresses. 3. Medical personnel--Congresses. 4. Health planning--Congresses.
I. Jaspers, Frans. II. Tarlov, Alvin R. III. Vrijland, Eric L. IV. European Symposium on Health Manpower Planning (1982 : University Limburg) V. Dutch Association of Junior Hospital Doctors. VI. Sveriges yngre läkares förening. VII. Rijksuniversiteit Limburg. Faculteit der Geneeskunde.
RA410.9.E86H4 1983 331.12'9161'094 82-24607

ISBN-13: 978-94-009-6695-6 e-ISBN-13: 978-94-009-6693-2
DOI: 10.1007/978-94-009-6693-2

Contents

Session I: Importance of Manpower Planning

Session II: Realities in Manpower Planning in Europe

Session III: Methods and Strategies in Manpower Planning

Preface

In most European countries there is a growing imbalance between the supply and demand of medical manpower. Though many national governments, international organizations and scientific institutes, and also, with a view from a different angle, doctors associations recognize this problem, it appears to be very difficult to bring all people concerned with this problem together in order to find a solution.

On this occasion, the initiative to arrange an international meeting was taken by the junior-doctors associations of The Netherlands and Sweden with the organizational support of the Faculty of Medicine of University Limburg, Maastricht, The Netherlands, and under the auspices of the Permanent Working Group of European Junior Hospital Doctors.

The symposium should be considered as a step in a series of continuing activities within the field of health manpower planning. The Organization for Economic Cooperation and Development (OECD) organized a working symposium on Long-Range Forecasting and Planning in 1968 (Bellaglio, Italy), followed by the Expert Committee of the OECD which produced the 'New Directives in Education for Changing Health Care System' (OECD-CERI report, Paris 1975).

The Dutch ministries of Education and Sciences and of Health and Environmental Protection organized a seminar on 'Cooperation of Health Care and Education at Regional Level, Responsibilities and Cost Allocation' (1978, Noordwijkerhout, The Netherlands). Following this, the Dutch Association of Junior Hospital Doctors (LVAG) organized a national conference 'Today a consultant in training, tomorrow an unemployed specialist?' (1980, Utrecht, The Netherlands).

The aims of this Symposium were to summarize the present situation as to the problem of health manpower in Europe and to attempt to develop a set of criteria and recommendations that can contribute to the search for a solution to these problems.

The growing imbalance between supply and demand of medical manpower is not merely a problem of numbers. Since the health industry is essentially labour-intensive, the planning of health manpower, a critical component, is also concerned with the type and quality of education, the workplace and the organization of health care.

Thus, the symposium was organized as a series of sessions whereby a discussion on a specific aspect of the problem was introduced by an invited expert. After these sessions the participants discussed in small workshops some specific aspects of the data and problems presented and helped to formulate the final conclusions and recommendations of the symposium.

With the publication of the Proceedings of the Symposium, the editors want to make an appeal to the many authorities, bodies and individuals to continue to seek the roads that will eventually lead to a practical and effective synchronizing of the supply and demand of medical manpower.

It would be impossible to give due thanks to everyone whose writings, endeavours and informal conversations have helped to organize the symposium and edit these proceedings. However, some exceptions have to be made. The editors wish to thank the organizations and industrial firms whose generous financial support primarily made possible the organization of the symposium and the publication of these proceedings.

All will be pleased to hear that the symposium was a great success.

Mrs Elsedien de Groot was the motor of the excellent administrative staff of the department of surgery of the Faculty of Medicine of the University Limburg, without whose help the organizational procedures would have failed. It wouldn't have been possible for us to write and speak the English language without the patient help of dr Mark Harvey, clinical chemist. Last but not least we owe a great deal to mrs Ans Steenbrink for typing the manuscripts and making them ready for the printer.

One agreement, made by the symposium, has not been added to the list of conclusions and recommendations published here. This was that the organizers were to publish the proceedings and recommendations of the symposium within four months. Unfortunately it took more time than was expected to collect and collate all the presented papers, to prepare and carry out the printing.

Planning is no business for amateurs!

Frans Jaspers
Alvin Tarlov
Eric Vrijland

INTRODUCTORY STATEMENTS

MINISTER
VAN VOLKSGEZONDHEID EN
MILIEUHYGIËNE

INTRODUCTION

From a government point of view, manpower planning is anything but simple. Even such a basic definition as "keeping a constant balance between the demand for qualified workers and their availability in sufficient numbers", demands virtually prophetic powers. Not only does government have to possess the required instruments if it is to adopt a specific manpower planning policy, but, in view of the long time needed to train new recruits and the length of a person's working life, it will have to make long-term forecasts of demand for professional workers and the potential workforce. The problems involved are very great and can only be solved in consultation with all the parties concerned - consumers, financiers and members of the professions. The various aspects which would have to be considered include:

- the development of a systematic structure for all the professions involved, including any new ones, and a suitable training system;
- an adequate information system on all those training for a career in health care, as well as on those already employed in the field;
- analysing the factors which influence the demand for health manpower;
- the development of suitable manpower planning instruments;
- the consequences a manpower planning policy may have for health care costs, the conditions of employment of the workers and other related factors.

This list is by no means exhaustive: no doubt many more subjects will be added after we have heard the wide range of speakers. What we should not lose sight of, however, in dealing with so many different aspects during the symposium, is that manpower planning is only a means to an end: ensuring that the patient or client is given counsel and care by people with a high standard of training and in sufficient numbers to fit them for their task.

Mrs. M.H.M.F. Gardeniers,
Minister of Health
and Environmental Protection.

MINISTER VAN ONDERWIJS EN WETENSCHAPPEN

INTRODUCTION

For an optimal functioning of the public health service an efficient coordination between the health system and vocational training is indispensable. In this respect both qualitative and quantitative aspects are relevant. One of the objectives of the Dutch government is the furthering of this proces.
In this era of limited financial means society can't afford any longer very specific and often prolonged vocational training of students in the knowledge of their future unemployment.
In view of this it is a good initiative of the Dutch Association of Junior Hospital Doctors to organize - in collaboration with The Swedish Association of Junior Hospital Doctors and The Faculty of Medicine of the University Limburg - a symposium on the subject of "Health Manpowerplanning : methods and strategies for maintenance of standards and cost-control".

The minister of education
and sciences,

drs. W.J. Deetman.

WORLD HEALTH ORGANIZATION

1211 GENEVA 27 - SWITZERLAND

ORGANISATION MONDIALE DE LA SANTÉ

1211 GENÈVE 27 - SUISSE

Planning health manpower for health for all by the year 2000

The European Symposium on Health Manpower Planning is considered to be an important event as it is meeting during a crucial period of the health development of humanity. With a historic resolution the 30th World Health Assembly in 1977 launched a movement for a New International Health Order by declaring that "the main social target of governments and WHO in the coming decades should be the attainment by all citizens of the world by the year 2000 of a level of health that will permit them to lead a socially and economically productive life".

In this concept health is a main component of quality of life, itself largely contributing to, and benefiting from, socioeconomic development. Thus the "main social target" of "health for all by the year 2000" is evidently a far-sounding echo of the New International Economic Order.

In 1978 an International Conference on Primary Health Care was held in Alma Ata, USSR, where governments of WHO Member States were represented at a high level. The Conference declared solemnly that "health for all by the year 2000" is a main social target and "primary health care is the key to attaining this target as a part of development in the spirit of social justice".

It is clearly understood that for a revolutionary goal there is a need for revolutionary policy and strategy in all fields of health development, health manpower not excluded.

It is evident that to achieve the goal set for the year 2000 there is a need to plan, train and deploy health manpower, in response to specific needs of people, as an integral part of the health infrastructure, both from the point of view of quality and of quantity.

The new health manpower development policies, principles, priorities, objectives and targets, reflecting this philosophy, are all based on the concept of integrated health services and health manpower development (HSMD).

In this concept of HSMD it is necessary to formulate national health manpower policies as part of national health policies which, in turn, are an integral part of national socioeconomic development policies and are based on the overall national political framework. Health manpower plans are then to be based on those policies and be integral elements of the general national socioeconomic, educational and manpower plans and based on the appreciation of local resources and needs. Health manpower planning, in this concept, consists in identifying and defining the categories, with their respective job descriptions,

.../-

numbers and ratios of health workers required for the development of health services, and the composition of the health teams, striking the balance among health team members that is best adapted to local conditions. Health manpower plans prepared on the basis of policies will define not only the numbers but also the categories and types of health personnel to be trained, and indicate the knowledge, skills and attitude, area and level of competence needed to carry out the tasks to be performed by each of them. The definition of job patterns, on the basis of functional analysis, for the different types of worker within the health team, will then lead to the specification of requirements and the translation of such requirements into learning objectives and subsequently into educational programmes, curricula, and methods (including evaluation instruments) to assist the learners in achieving those objectives.

Health manpower plans conceived on the basis of the "health for all" concept serve as a guidance for the training and management components of the health manpower development process as well.

Clearly, the "health for all" concept has major implications for all components of the health manpower development process, for planning, training and utilization of health personnel in all their interdependence. This Symposium can, and certainly will, substantially contribute to the further clarification of all these implications and, through this, to the achievement of health for all. WHO therefore, is most interested in its deliberations, as well as in the outcome and practical implications of those deliberations, and will follow them with the attention they certainly merit.

T. Fülöp, M.D.
Director, Division of
Health Manpower Development

The World Bank / 1818 H Street, N.W., Washington, D.C. 20433, U.S.A. • Telephone: (202) 477-1234 • Cables: INTBAFRAD

INTRODUCTION

The success of investments in productive capacity or infrastructure, which dominate the lending of international aid agencies such as the World Bank, depends heavily upon the availability of trained manpower at all levels to ensure their continued efficient operation. We are acutely aware of this need and endeavor either to include in our lending arrangements provision for the necessary training, or at least to be satisfied that manpower with the requisite skills is available, and that the terms and conditions of employment are such as to facilitate recruitment. Thus, although education and health projects per se form a relatively small proportion of total World Bank lending, human resource development is a central objective of our operations.

The health sector poses a particular challenge. Compared with investments in most other fields, the recurrent costs of operation and maintenance of facilities are extremely high in the health sector, and these costs are dominated by salaries and wages of health personnel. Problems are compounded in developing countries in that trained health workers tend to be in abundant supply where least needed, and non-existent where health needs are most acute; and training is often inappropriate to address the major health priorities.

The symposium on Health Manpower Planning, while concentrating on conditions and policies in developed countries, nevertheless addresses a subject, the principles of which are of universal relevance. We hope that it helps to stimulate further debate and analysis of this critical subject.

Dr. John R. Evans
Director
Population, Health & Nutrition Department
The World Bank
Washington, D. C.

OPENING SESSION

Welcome Address and Introduction

E.L. Vrijland, M.D.

In dutch 'hartelijk welkom' and in english a sincere welcome to this European Symposium on Health Manpower Planning in Maastricht.

I like to direct a special welcome to the Minister of Health and Environmental Protection of The Netherlands, a representative of the ministry of Education and Sciences of The Netherlands and our hosts, the Dean of the Medical Faculty and Chairman of the Board of Governers of the State University Limburg, and the Mayor of the city of Maastricht. I would also like to welcome the Director of the Division of Manpower Development of the World Health Organization, the Chairman of the Royal Dutch Medical Association, the Presidents of the Dutch as well as the Swedish Medical Associations of Junior Hospital Doctors and the Coordinating Secretary of the Permanent Working Group of European Junior Hospital Doctors.

Let me try to give you a resumé of how the idea to hold this seminar came about. Slowly but surely (almost) everybody who has anything to do with health services, or training health service employees, has begun to realize that by the normal criteria there is an overproduction of doctors in the highly industrialized countries. This stems from the fact that the supply of doctors and medical specialists is not coordinated with the needs of the society, and has led to – literally – doctors 'on the dole'. In turn this is leading to disruption of the 'division of labour' within the health service, in that doctors seek employment for which they are overqualified; it leads to destruction of the investment capital and can eventually bring about a lowering of the quality of health care through the loss of skill and experience.

In The Netherlands, the Dutch Association of Junior Hospital Doctors organized in 1980 a conference 'Today consultant in training, tomorrow unemployed specialist?', in which special attention was given to the question as to 'how' and 'to what extent' has the system of supply and demand led to unemployment among doctors.

The role of medical education within the health service was also discussed. The Association of Junior Hospital Doctors wishes to develop the foundations laid down by this conference and in particular to broaden the scope of the discussion to a pan-European level.

Right from its conception in 1974, an independent working group of young European Hospital Doctors, the PWG, recognized the importance of this transnational medical manpower problem. The PWG has since then, through the collection and publication of information, tried to stimulate the international organizations and national governments, responsible for policymaking, into action.

With the enactment of the EEC directives in 1976, which among other things regulated inter-EEC recognition of medical degrees, any member-doctor can, in principle, without restriction, practise medicine anywhere within the Community. Thus from that moment discussion of the man-power problem became supra-national and pan-European.

An interesting study of this problem was produced through the initiatives of the Swedish Junior Hospital Doctors Association, which has not only stimulated the discussion internationally, but has also led to the formulation of prospective legislation in Sweden, to align the supply of doctors with the demand.

Thus, through a merging of ideas within the organizations mentioned, the plan to hold this conference was born. This was based on the need to contribute to, and further the development of methods and strategies for manpower planning that would be useful for the european industrialized countries.

Plans have to be effected. The organization must function as a well run sewing machine. The organizing committee was therefore overjoyed when the State University Limburg, and in particular the department of surgery, offered to take a major part of the organization upon itself. It should be mentioned that the State University Limburg is noted for the fact that it feels responsible for not only the medical technical education of its trainee-doctors, but also for how these trainees fit into the society as practising clinicians. Thus this symposium fits in well with the philosophy of this new university.

Who do we want to reach? What kind of audience do we hope for? In the first place, of course, the people who are actually busy with, or will be involved in manpower planning within the health service. For example, national and provincial administrators, representatives of other, for example financially concerned groups, such as health insurers, hospitals, medical, paramedical, nursing and ancillary health care professions and of course, last but not least individuals from all the professions within the health service. I am pleased to be able to say that representatives of all these groups are here today, or at least have sent their registration fees in.

As you can see from the programme we have obviously had to limit the number and scope of subjects that we can handle. This has visibly resulted in a programme orientated from the viewpoint of the hospital doctor.

Minister, ladies and gentlemen,

we are only too well aware that we have created an extremely tight schedule which will demand a lot from you the coming few days. I hope that you have not come to Maastricht for nothing and that this symposium will result in a series of worthwhile conclusions and recommendations which will lead to real measures being taken to solve all or at least some of the problems which face our health services today.

Official Opening of the Symposium by the Minister of Health and Environmental Protection of The Netherlands

Mrs M.H.M.F. Gardeniers

Mr chairman, ladies and gentlemen,

Firstly, may I say how much I appreciate the invitation to open this symposium today. I am particularly happy to do so because your subject for discussion over the next two days is one which is becoming increasingly topical. There is growing pressure for manpower planning in the health services, and I believe that the main reasons are as follows.

First and most important is the rise in unemployment among those who have trained for jobs in the health services. In view of the number of students currently training for such jobs, the discrepancy between the supply of qualified staff and the demand for their services can be expected to increase still further in the next few years.

Secondly, there are the attempts made by the Government to control and limit the growth and cost of the health services. With budgets becoming tighter, it is important to make the best possible use of manpower.

The third and final reason why manpower planning is called for is the danger that future health service staff may not acquire the skills, knowledge and attitudes they need in order to carry out their work. Since the quality of training largely determines the quality of health care, it is important that it should come up to proper professional standards. Although other reasons will no doubt be discussed in the course of the symposium, I shall confine my remarks to these three.

With regard to the discrepancy between the supply of qualified health care staff and the demand for their services, it is equally serious whether there is a surplus or a shortage. A surplus of staff can easily lead to the performance of tasks which are either unnecessary or unnecessarily complicated, and it is not impossible to imagine a situation where the best possible treatment is given but is then continued when it might be better to terminate it. In addition, the possible loss of skills and routine resulting from a surplus will do equally little to improve quality.

Shortages are no less of a problem. If there are not enough staff, the patient may not receive sufficient attention, and waiting lists may build up.

Surpluses or shortages are not only undesirable as far as the quality of health care is concerned; they are also unwelcome from the point of view of those being trained. If too many people are trained, some of them will discover that although they have studied for years they have no opportunity to practise their skills, or at best that they have to wait before they can do so. If on the other hand too few people are trained, they will discover that the demand for their services is too great and that they are overworked, which may lead to illness, absenteeism and a high turnover of the staff or premature departure from the profession.

An imbalance between the supply of professionally qualified staff and the demand for their services is also a source of dissatisfaction for the government. Investment in training holds few attractions if there is a likelihood that those being trained are going to find it difficult or impossible to get a job. If on the other hand there are staff shortages the government will find it difficult to guarantee the individual's right to health care.

The question is how manpower planning can help prevent such imbalances in the field of health care in the future. The purpose of manpower planning is to keep supply and demand in equilibrium, qualitatively as well as quantitatively. It is an attempt to create a situation where the right number of people have the right skills and attitudes in the right place at the right time. This requires a knowledge of the demand for health facilities and an ability to translate this into the demand for different categories of personnel. Information on the numbers of existing staff and on those being trained is also a requirement, as are methods of influencing the situation.

Meeting these requirements is no easy matter. Past experience would suggest that it is almost impossible, partly on account of the many factors outside the planner's control.

A system of planning so perfect as to prevent any future imbalance is, in my opinion, unattainable. I expect we do all agree on this. However, any plan is better than no plan at all, and some measures of timely control, however imperfect, can make a situation less serious than it would be if there were none at all and may obviate the necessity for ad hoc measures.

Control can be exercized in a number of ways, one of the most important being to regulate the number of people trained. This poses a problem in that, in-service training aside, training for a profession is not the sole aim of education. If greater emphasis is placed on other aims and less on the anticipated demands of the employment market, there will continue to be imbalances.

It must also be borne in mind that the employment market is to some extent international. If one country gears its capacity for training students to the demand for qualified manpower while another does not, the movement of labour from one country to another will create imbalances. There is thus a case for concluding international agreements on measures of this kind.

Other considerations apart, the possible lack of coordination between staff supply and demand may result in measures being taken to regulate who actually practises for example by restricting admission to a profession. This may be done for two reasons: to achieve a balanced distribution of staff throughout the country and to cope with the problem of oversupply. Restriction on entry is achieved in a number of ways; these include fixing the number of practices of a particular type in a particular region; controlling the issue of licences to persons and institutions where they are employed; and making the expansion of facilities, and therefore the increase in staff, subject to conditions. Entry to a profession can also be restricted by laying down requirements for job applicants, for example as regards qualifications.

In addition to regulating entry to a profession, measures can be taken to influence the supply of manpower available. These include making it easier for people to work part-time; shortening the working week; early retirement; lengthening or shortening the period of training; taking people into employment; and making changes in responsibilities and the way time at work is spent. Some of these measures will be taken on account of general trends in the employment situation rather than as a means of controlling the health care sector itself.

Apart from controlling the potential number of people employed, manpower planning can involve influencing demand for health care. For example, increasing the cover provided by insurance would increase demand, and therefore improve employment prospects as well. On the other hand, if patients were required to pay part of the cost of treatment themselves this would inevitably have the opposite effect. These two examples illustrate methods of dealing with either surpluses or shortages.

As you can imagine, since the government is attempting to limit and control the growth and cost of the health services, it does not advocate boosting demand for facilities. This does not mean that nothing new can be done, but it does mean that any new activities must be accommodated within the existing budget. In practice it means constantly reconsidering the work currently performed by the health services and placing the emphasis on improving efficiency and effectiveness. The effect this will have on jobs in the future is difficult to determine, although it is a factor that will have to be borne in mind when manpower requirements are planned and some kind of estimate will therefore have to be made, albeit only in the most general terms.

The mention of new activities brings me to the third reason for manpower planning I mentioned earlier: discrepancies between what qualified staff have learned and what they require in practice developments in health make constant new demands on the education system, and if it does not keep pace, professional standards will suffer. There is no point in teaching outdated skills, for example.

Manpower planning should include a consideration of the qualitative aspect of the relationship between education and employment. It helps a great deal if the medical profession is systematically structured to link up with the education system, thus preventing qualitative discrepancies as far as possible.

Mr chairman, ladies and gentlemen,

manpower planning in the health services is a complex subject, and a great many factors need to be taken into account. I have touched upon only a few, and there are many more I could add such as demography, epidemiology, medico-technical and cultural aspects, and so on. They will all affect demand for health care, the number and type of staff employed and the supply of qualified staff. All these aspects, and a few more besides, will no doubt come up for discussion during the conference. Much will be said about the advantages and disadvantages, and the possibilities and impossibilities, of manpower planning. Its international aspects will no doubt receive full attention, since we have among us speakers and participants from abroad. It will not be easy to find solutions or make concrete practical recommendations, but I hope that you will be able to come to some agreement on the subject. In the field of health care demand is mainly determined by supply, including the supply of personnel, market forces simply do not apply. Methods of control are therefore required. Your discussions should indicate the best methods of manpower planning and employment in the medical profession.

May I conclude by wishing you a very successful conference.

Planning Health Manpower for Health for All by the Year 2000

T. Fülöp, M.D.

It is a great pleasure for me to participate in this symposium which certainly meets in a crucial period of health development of humanity. The international health collaboration which started, in an organized form, in the middle of the last century has, if we may say so, come of age with the historic victory over smallpox. This has very clearly proved that with peaceful collaboration humanity is able to set and achieve targets which may seem difficult or, for some, even impossible to achieve.

The accumulated experience in international collaboration in general and in the health field especially, the conquest of smallpox, the great decision of the United Nations to set into motion a programme of action for the establishment of a new international economic order, the increasing realization of the great and growing inequities in health field were some of the main factors which conditioned a historic resolution of the 30th World Health Assembly in May 1977. This resolution after saying that 'faced with the magnitude of health problems and the inadequate and intolerably inequitable distribution of health resources throughout the world today' and 'considering that health is a basic human right and a world-wide social goal, and that it is essential to the satisfaction of basic human needs and the quality of life' and, 'reaffirming that the ultimate constitutional objective of WHO is the attainment by all people of the highest possible level of health', declared that 'the main social target of governments and WHO in the coming decades should be the attainment by all citizens of the world by the year 2000 of a level of health that will permit them to lead a socially and economically productive life'. (1)

In this concept health is a main component of quality of life, itself largely contributing to, and benefiting from, socio-economic development. Thus the 'main social target' of 'health for all by the year 2000' is evidently a far-sounding echo of the New International Economic Order, declaring in fact a New International Health Order. It stems from the recognition of the fact that health and socio-economic development are inseparable, and that health development can no longer be considered as the affair of the traditionally defined health sector alone, but should be the concern of all other interested development sectors, and thus it is of a truly intersectoral character.

Of course it is clearly understood that health for all is *not* a single, finite target: it is rather a process leading to progressive improvement in the health of people. The concept of health for all in this process will be interpreted and adapted differently by each country in the light of its social, economic and even political characteristics, the health status and morbidity patterns of its population, and the state of development of its health system. It is a moving target: as a certain health status is reached, people will set a target to reach a higher level, and so on. However, it is now a common understanding that 'there is a base-line below which no individuals in any country should find themselves' and 'by the year 2000, *all* people in *all* countries should have a level of health that will permit them to lead a socially and economically productive life'. What does this imply? 'The level of health of all people should be at least such that they are capable of working productively and of participating actively in the social life of the community in which they live'. (2)

Health for all is certainly a realistic concept. It 'does not mean that in the year 2000 doctors and nurses will provide medical care for everybody in the world for all their existing ailments; nor does it mean that in the year 2000 nobody will be sick or disabled. It does mean that health begins at home, in schools and in factories. It is there, where people live and work, that health is made or broken. It does mean that people will use better approaches than they do now for preventing disease and alleviating unavoidable disease and disability, and have better ways of growing up, growing old and dying gracefully.

It does mean that there will be an even distribution of whatever resources for health are available. It does mean that essential health care will be accessible to *all* individuals and families in an acceptable and affordable way, and with their full involvement. And it does mean that people will realize that they themselves have the power to shape their lives and the lives of their families, free from the avoidable burden of disease, and aware that ill-health is not inevitable'. (3)

In essence this means freedom from avoidable suffering, pain, disability and death for all people by the year 2000 and altogether a different approach whereby health is considered in the broader context of its contribution to, and promotion by, social and economic development.

In September 1978, an International Conference of Primary Health Care was held in Alma Ata, USSR, where governments of WHO Member States were represented at a high level. The Conference declared solemnly that 'health for all by the year 2000' is a main social target and 'primary health care is the key to attaining this target as a part of development in the spirit of social justice'. (4)

In 1979 the Health Assembly endorsed the Alma Ata Report and Declaration and invited Member States to act individually in formulating national strategies and collectively in formulating regional and global strategies. In response to that invitation, Member States of WHO formulated their national strategies for 'health for all by the year 2000' as broad lines of action required in all sectors to give effect to the new health policy. Based on these national strategies, and in support of them, regional and finally global strategies were worked out.

The Global Strategy for Health for All by the Year 2000 was discussed and adopted by the 34th World Health Assembly in May 1981. It reflects the national and regional strategies as seen from a global perspective. It is not a separate 'WHO strategy', but an expression of individual and collective national responsibility, and of ways and means, and a plan of action, to support it by WHO.

The 'health for all' concept and the Global Strategy, are global in a number of different senses of this term. One obvious dimension of globality is that it equally refers to and is valid for both develop*ed* and develop*ing* countries. Discussing the world health and related socioeconomic problems and trends, the Global Strategy emphatically points out the serious health problems of developed countries. These problems are, of course, wellknown but you may permit me to list them here: cardiovascular diseases, cancer, accidents, environmental health problems due to industrialization and urbanization, mental disorders to the extent that vast numbers live on tranquillizers, social pathology such as alcohol, nicotine and drug abuse, high suicide rates, lung cancer and other chronic diseases due to smoking, obesity due to overeating, chronic diseases and other socio-medical problems related to old age – and all these are growing.

Even health services are not free of problems: the overwhelming proportion of resources for the delivery of health care is concentrated in the large cities; these resources are devoted to expensive, highly sophisticated technology, unduly emphasizing the curative element, more often than not useful only to a very small fragment of the population; undue emphasis on secondary and on tertiary care to the detriment of the often quite rudimentary primary care; altogether a deep fragmentation of health care which is mainly provided to the individual, largely neglecting the community with its needs and the real objective of health services, which is the improvement of the health of the entire population; the absence of well formulated health policy and plans, and of coordination both within the health sector and with other sectors of socioeconomic development and a lack of a coherent health system, institutions functioning in a more or less unrelated way; the lack of involvement of the community, i.e. of the 'consumers', in the planning, provision and evaluation of health services; even in the most highly developed countries the explosive costs of health care make it impossible to provide the complete range of health technology to the whole population although social pressures are demanding this even when it is not really necessary. Finally, we may mention here, as it is so relevant to the topic of our symposium, the lack of proper planning of health personnel and, hence, the spectre of over-production of certain categories, e.g. the recently so much talked of plethora of doctors.

It is quite evident therefore that developed countries, as well as developing ones, will strive for 'health for all' and they too stand to benefit from international cooperation in their struggle. The strategy lists areas where such cooperation will foreseeably be intensified and collaboration in the field ofhealth services and health manpower development, primarily in the form of promotion of critical analysis and exchange of experiences could also be added to the list.

Further the strategy is 'global' also from the point of view of trying to review the 'globality' of the problems to be solved to attain 'health for all'. It is clearly understood that for a revolutionary goal there is a need for revolutionary policy and strategy in all fields of health development, health manpower not excluded.

It is evident that to achieve the goal set for the year 2000 there is a need to plan, train and deploy health manpower in response to specific needs of people as an integral part of the health infrastructure, both from the point of view of quality and of quantity.

The new health manpower development policies, principles, priorities, objectives and targets, reflecting this philosophy, are all based on the concept of integrated *h*ealth *s*ervices and health *m*anpower *d*evelopment (HSMD). This concept has been very actively promoted in the past few years. It means that the quality *and* quantity of health manpower has to be planned in response to the specific needs of the national health system and, through this, to the health needs and demands of the population. Then health personnel should be trained according to these plans with a view to 'placing at the disposal of the system the right kind of manpower in the right numbers at the right time in the right place'. This training should also 'ensure that health workers are socially motivated and provided with the necessary incentives to serve communities'. (5)

Management of health personnel should thus ensure that personnel planned and trained in view of *needs* will be most efficiently deployed to meet those needs, and obtain job satisfaction by satisfying the health needs and demands of people they are meant to serve. An effective monitoring system would provide feedback data on which to base the adjustment of planning and 'production' of health personnel. The self-directing, cybernetic circle of the health manpower development process (planning, 'production' and management of health personnel), created this way, has to be entirely geared to, and in fact integrated with, the process of health services development.

In this concept of HSMD it is necessary to formulate national health manpower policies as part of national health which, in turn, are an integral part of national socio-economic development policies and are based on the overall national political framework. Health manpower plans are then to be based on those policies and be integral elements of the general national socio-economic, educational and manpower plans and based on the appreciation of local resources and needs. Health manpower planning, in this concept, consists in identifying and defining the categories, numbers and ratios of health workers required, and the composition of the health teams, striking the balance among health team members that is best adapted to local conditions. Health manpower plans prepared on the basis of policies will define not only the numbers but also the categories and types of health personnel to be trained, and indicate the knowledge, skills and attitude, area and level of competence needed to carry out the tasks to be performed by each of them. The definition of job patterns, on the basis of functional analysis, for the different types of workers within the health team, will then lead to the specification of requirements and the translation of such requirements into learning objectives and subsequently into educational programmes, curricula, and methods (including evaluation instruments) to assist the learners in achieving those objectives.

Health manpower plans conceived on the basis of the 'health for all' concept serve as a guidance for the training component of the health manpower development process as well. Training programmes that are planned with this most important social target in mind, aiming at competencies relevant to its achievement, will tend to be

- competency based
- community oriented and
- community based
- multiprofessional
- integrated on a problem-basis
- student-centred (self-learning oriented), and
- adapted to the development of sciences and to local needs and resources.

There are an increasing number of programmes which follow these principles, among them the Faculty of Medicine of the University Limburg. In 1979 a number of those programmes formed, under WHO sponsorship, a Network of Community Oriented Educational Institutions for Health Sciences, of which the central secretariat is here in Maastricht under the most able leadership of Dean Greep.

Efforts to plan and train health manpower loose much of their value if the trained personnel is not used to best advantage by the health services. Indeed, shortage of personnel may in some instances be related to the fact that existing manpower is not being properly used. Not even developed countries can afford to waste their highly trained health manpower, but the economic use of personnel is particularly essential in less developed countries.

Optimal utilization of health personnel demands that available health manpower is distributed within the country – and within the different sectors of the health services – in direct relation to the needs of the population; no member of the health team carries out activities that could be performed by less qualified personnel, on the principle of using the smallest volume of skill or group of skills with the necessary related knowledge to perform a specified job; and that all health activities should be undertaken at the most peripheral level of the health services as is practicable, by the workers most *suitably* trained to carry out these activities; the interest of each member of the health services is stimulated by providing motivation and incentives, such as conditions that give the worker a feeling of responsibility and a consciousness that his work is useful, effective, and contributing to the general development of the community, an appropriate system of social security, as well as moral and financial recognition of achievement, based on systematic review of living and working conditions and achievements; a system of continuing education that will provide opportunities for each member of the health team, and stimulate him to maintain and improve his performance in relation to the health needs of the population; job satisfaction and security of tenure for all staff, whatever their level, within a properly organized career structure, with fair advancement, possibilities for promotion, with vertical and horizontal mobility, including access to posts with increasing responsibility; and that each health worker receives constant technical support and supervision within a participatory system of teams at all levels, as needed.

If all the above conditions are fulfilled, conditions for the proper management of health personnel will be present; and, if well administered, a sufficient quantity and quality of health personnel will not only be attracted to posts in health services where they are needed but will also stay as long as they are needed.

Clearly, the 'health for all' concept has major implications for all components of the health manpower development process, for planning, training and utilization of health personnel in all their interdependence.

On the basis of the definition of the policies and strategies for health manpower development in general and of health manpower planning especially, the main thrusts in health manpower development for the foreseeable future have been worked out.

First and foremost there is a need to foster national political will to change all that needs changing in human resources development to achieve health for all by the year 2000 through primary health care. That also means to emphasize the relevance, i.e. the 'what for' aspect of action, in addition to the traditional methodological, i.e. 'how' aspect, e.g. in such areas as the manpower planning, teacher training, etc. Change also means shift in emphasis in content, where needed, e.g. to stress the quality aspects of manpower plans, their relevance to needs, their feasibility and especially their utilization, implementation instead of just promoting the preparation of plans (often irrelevant and largely unused).

As to the different subsystems of the health manpower development process, it is a general agreement that much more emphasis than in the past should be placed on, and more attention given to, manpower planning, including problems of oversupply and imbalances, as well as manpower management and utilization, in addition to the classical stress on 'production'. In the latter field training of, support to, and monitoring of, health workers in and for primary care, along with the development of task-and problem-based community-oriented education programmes for all categories of health workers, physicians, of course, included. Finally, national research in the human resources field is needed to provide a scientifically sound basis for the decisions that will have to be made concerning the changes needed.

Concluding, we may state that the key to further progress in the health manpower development field, in terms of the goal 'health for all by the year 2000 through primary health care', is *the promotion of national political will to seek out and apply the right solutions to well-diagnosed priority problems*. There seems to be a *health challenge* here *to which a right political*, and unequivocal political, *response is needed*. It seems therefore that priority should now be given, at least for a while, to the stimulation of national political will and the appropriate technical approaches and solutions should all be subordinated to the clearly set main targets supported by that firm national will.

The key-word in the future should be *relevance*. A systematic, integrated and holistic programme approach will have to be applied with relevance as the main aspect of all activities - relevance to the main social target of health for all by the year 2000, and in fact, to the health needs and demands of the people. In view of this, the three main output indicators of the health manpower development process for the future might be:

a) extension of health coverage with special regard to primary health care;
b) improvement of quality of health coverage;
c) community participation and satisfaction.

Health for all by the year 2000 is the biggest health challenge humanity ever set for itself. It *is* a realistic aim but there is a long way to go to achieve it even in the most developed countries. There is an implication in it for all elements of society and among them for the universities and health personnel teaching institutions. This presentation has tried to throw some light on these implications also, and hopes only to provoke discussion which will then lead to further clarification of the role of those and other institutions concerned and to their closer association with this world-wide and ever larger movement, which aims at health for all by the year 2000 through primary health care.

With these thoughts may I wish you, on behalf of the World Health Organization and myself, fruitful deliberations that bring us all closer to the solution of your problems and, through this, to our great common goal: health for all.

References:

1. Handbook of resolutions and decisions of the World Health Assembly and the Executive Board, Vol. II, Fourth edition (1973-1980), WHO, Geneva, 1981, p. 1.
2. Global Strategy for Health for All by the Year 2000, WHO, Geneva, 1981 ('Health for All' Series, No. 3), p. 31.
3. Ibid., pp. 31-32.
4. Alma Ata 1978. Primary Health Care, WHO, Geneva, 1978 ('Health for All' Series, No. 1), p. 3.
5. As footnote (2), but p. 45.

Welcome Address by the Coordinating Secretary of the Permanent Working Group of European Junior Hospital Doctors (PWG)

A. Seiler, M.D.

This European Symposium on Health Manpower Planning will be held under the auspices of the Permanent Working Group of European Junior Hospital Doctors, PWG.

What is the PWG?

The PWG represents an organized and coordinated collaboration between organizations including junior hospital doctors in Belgium, Denmark, Finland, France, Iceland, Ireland, Italy, The Netherlands, Portugal, Spain, Sweden, Switzerland, the United Kingdom and Western Germany.

During the last two years contacts have been established with organizations in Austria, Greece and Norway.

After four years of preparation PWG was founded in 1976 in Western Germany. The PWG include both EEC and non-EEC countries in view of its broad European nature, but a subcommittee of the EEC was establised in 1977 as the PWG realized that an EEC identity was necessary in relation to the developments within the EEC, and the PWG has therefore also recognized THE STANDING COMMITTEE OF DOCTORS OF THE EEC as the leading organization of the profession within the EEC area.

In the constitution of PWG we read, that the Permanent Working Group is open to one national delegation from each European country. The delegation shall represent recognized national organizations of junior hospital doctors. A junior hospital doctor is defined as a doctor at hospital, at a university institution, or in a training position related to these, who has not yet attained a final post of independent practice within the Health Services of his country.

The aims of the Permanent Working Group are:

- to improve the relationships between junior hospital doctors in the European countries,
- to exchange informations on and develop a common approach to problems of mutual interest, such as medical education, specialist training and working conditions,
- to improve and protect the standards of total health care in Europe, and
- to further the professional interests of junior hospital doctors on a European level.

The work of PWG is done in several subcommittees, so in

- the subcommittee on working conditions and vacant posts for foreign doctors in the European countries,
- the subcommittee on postgraduate training and specialist medical education,
- the subcommittee on manpower, production and needs,
- the EEC-subcommittee.

According to the decisions taken by the PWG-meetings, subcommittees shall be formed to work on special items.

At the beginning the highest priority in the working programme of the PWG was the promotion of a broader European educational market for hospital doctors training at specialist level. The purposes of such a system were elaborated in 1978 in a Memorandum on temporary migration and include:

- promote the spread of medical knowledge between the European countries on the old principle 'learning by doing' - and using the professional individual as a transport medium for communications,
- further European medical research by creating an educational flow of hospital doctors between clinical institutions with the same research areas in several countries, and
- further European integration by giving a professional group the opportunity to see how their colleagues think and work in other European countries.

The interest among doctors for further medical education outside their own cultural circles has existed throughout history. So the Italian Lanfranchi (± 1315) carried with him a unique surgical tradition from Bologna to Paris. The English John Harvey (1578-1658) - who discovered the blood circulation - studied for a long time in Padua, Italy. The French Ambroise Paré (1510-1564) gained most of his surgical skill on the battle fields of Europe in contact with colleagues from many nations. The Dutch Vesalius (1514-1564) started his famous anatomical studies in Paris. The Danish Niels Stensen - who discovered the essential details of several glands - studied during his life time (1638-1686) in Amsterdam, Leyden, Paris, Montpellier and Florence. The Swiss Theophrastus Pompastus Paracelsus from Hohenheim - who perhaps more than anybody else in his time associated practice with theoretical medicine - was most of his life a wandering scholar in Europe.

That's history. - And we, today, what shall we do?

I think, that the time is now due for Europe to take over the tradition which developed after 1945 of European doctors undertaking postgraduate training and studies in the USA.

For this propose we need a manpower planning in Europe. The PWG has a good eye for the needs of the present time and the future. Years before this actual symposium on Health Manpower Planning PWG studied the question related to the overproduction of medical doctors in Europe. Last year we defined the positions of unemployed, underemployed, misemployed, underpayed and overqualified doctors.

All members of PWG hope that this symposium can clarify the present situation of health manpower. We all hope, that we are able to develop a set of criteria and recommendations that can contribute to the search for a solution of the main problem of our profession in Europe: health manpower planning.

SESSION I:

IMPORTANCE OF MANPOWER PLANNING

Manpower Planning as an European Problem and as a Task for Europe: the Need for International Legislation

W. Albeda, Ph.D.

Higher education has expanded very rapidly during the last thirty years. As Mark Blang remarked several years ago authorities apparently had the notion that something like Say's Law operates in markets for professional manpower, supply creating its own demand. (1) Educational planning was until comparatively recent time rather haphazard in character and was concerned with individual educational institutions rather than with entire educational systems.

The post-war interest in manpower planning using the planning of education as a tool stemmed from different sources. There was a first wave of interest, from which we inherited many interesting studies on the economics of education, inspired by the concerns of Western governments with the development of economic growth. Partly as a consequence of the Sputnik-experience, partly inspired by studies like that of F. Denison on the relationship between education and economic growth, governments wanted to expand their higher education as one element in the race between East and West that seemed to take place mainly in the field of comparative growth rates. Making a study of the sources of the growth of income per person employed Denison came to the famous conclusion that improved education of the labour force constituted an amount equal to 42% of the total increase in national income per person employed. Investment in education seemed to be one of the most promising roads to higher economic growth. As a consequence the educational system was treated by governments even more friendly than was already the case. It appears to be reasonable to expect that given an increase of the National Income per head, education will anyhow experience an increase of interest. In this sense education has the character of a consumption: the population will spend more money on education even more than proportionally with the growth of the National Income. In this sense the interest of the citizens as consumers of education went into the same direction as the interest of governments embarked upon the project of increasing economic growth.

Since the golden sixties, the economic outlook has changed dramatically. The present depression not only put an end to expectations of rapid economic growth. The modern welfare state, with its in general high social security outlays, high expenditure on social services, health and education, reacts in an understandable way to the depression. The total expenditure, especially as regards social security and the social services increases dramatically. At the same time the inherent trend in government expenditure goes on. As a consequence all governments find themselves confronted with substantial and growing deficits in their budgets. These deficits not only do not lead to the reestablishment of economic growth, they strengthen the present inflation and thereby increase unemployment: Keynes' built-in stabilizers have become destabilizers.

As a consequence the present interest in manpower and educational planning is much more so than 11 years ago inspired by the necessity of limiting the explosive expansion of government expenditure.

Already at the end of the sixties the OECD expressed its concern about the increase of government expenditure in the three sectors, education, health and welfare. These sectors not only have a growing government expenditure in common, but also a number of other characteristics: they are rather labour intensive, they employ highly qualified manpower and have only limited possibilities for an increase of productivity. Moreover they possess an inherent tendency to growth. At that time these sectors were singled out by the OECD as the sectors governments should concentrate on, if they wish to put a limit to their expenditure. Now as a consequence of the growth of unemployment and other forms of non-activity these sectors are joined by social security and social services in general. No government can under the present circumstances leave the development of these sectors and more particularly the development of the health sector to the outcome of the process of almost autonomous growth that we have seen since 1950. One very important element in this concern of course is the development of a firm manpower planning.

Not only governments are interested in manpower planning. As the goal of reaching full employment is receding behind the horizon of slower economic growth the people working in the sectors most threatened by surplusses of manpower and thus by unemployment and lower income perspectives ask themselves whether timely action may prevent both threats. Perhaps I might say that the present congress is an example of the way in which Junior Hospital Doctors react to this new state of affairs.

Some remarks on manpower planning

The need for manpower planning arises as a consequence of the shortcomings of the working of the price mechanism on the labour market. These shortcomings are wellknown: lack of transparency of the market, the market is a short term mechanism that cannot take account of long term perspectives and so on.

I think that expecially the fact that the education of highly educated manpower takes a rather long time, leads governments and the people working in the health services to look upon manpower planning as an instrument. What do they want to achieve by manpower planning?

Everybody agrees that the final goal of manpower planning should be to establish a balance between demand and supply for the different types of professions and skills.

I want to make two preliminary remarks with regard to the goals of manpower planning.

We have to distinguish between on the one hand the effective demand for health services and what could be called the *need* for the health services. The effective demand and the final need are not necessarily the same.

'Need' is a very difficult concept. As one American observer puts it: 'An increasingly professionalized, socialized and organized structure satisfies what the professional conceives as needs'. (2) There is no single concept of need and, as Kenneth Building remarks, especially no single concept of need for health services. One's demand for medical care is what the patient wants; his need for medical care is what the doctor thinks he ought to have. 'It is dangerous to go from' analogous statements about needs, representing expressions of social aspirations or expectations, to statements about 'Demand', representing descriptions of labour-market situations, to statements about the 'requirements' of manpower and other resources for satisfying needs at a given level under unspecified conditions of utilization. This quotation from Henry David seems to me very relevant for our present considerations about manpower planning in the health services.

The search for criteria proves to be a rather frustrating activity.. What about personnel-to-population ratios? Is it acceptable to compare the different ratios and then to calculate the potential need for medical manpower by bringing all geographic areas below some selected standard ratio (based f.i. on the average for all regions) up to it? It is clear that this method always will find that a shortage exists.

The economist of course will turn his attention to the market and will try to find out what is happening with regard to the incomes level of the personnel concerned. Is it increasing? That would be a clear indication that there is a shortage. Is it decreasing? That is a clear indication that there is a certain amount of overdoctoring.

Some economists would like to see a constant surplus of physicians as an assurance of access to one when needed. Others favor a taut supply, on the ground that physicians are able to generate a demand for their services when hard-pressed financially.

Economists furthermore will warn against the danger to look upon manpower planning for one medical profession isolated from the other professions: as comparative studies from different countries even within the limited space of the Common Market, show different countries have different ratios between the number of specialists, physicians and nurses. We should go further and realize that the medical professions are no islands. Developments in other sectors may influence both the demand and the supply side for medical personnel.

Mr President,

It is not my intention to trespass into the territory that other speakers have agreed to cover. However, it seems to me that the question that I have to deal with: the need for international legislation, cannot be dealt with, if we do not see the uncertainties and pitfalls that surround us when we venture into this field. In the present situation the whole context of our discussion is dictated by the basic factor of the financial crisis in all modern welfare states that I mentioned before. To my knowledge no European country finds itself in the situation where the government can just look at the development of, say, the last twenty five year and extrapolate the findings for the coming ten or twenty years. For the time being the basic factor determining manpower planning for the medical sector is not the need for medical care however defined, but the expected possibility for the State to finance the development of this sector. Governments will tend to determine first the maximum percentage of their national income they want to spend on medical care, to derive from the resulting figure the need or requirement for medical manpower as it is composed of the different professions.

In that sense our problem (in a more or less barbaric way, using the yardstick of the budgetary space) is simplified somewhat. We need not dwell too much on the uncertainties of needs and expectations. That problem is solved for us by politicians who, faced by increasing budget deficits have to solve their own impossible problem: how to divide the limited means at their disposal between sectors so different and incomparable as health, education, defence, public transport, roadbuilding, housing, and so on.

Given the result of that impossible, but necessary exercitation, manpower planning becomes a necessity and a possibility. *It is a necessity* for two reasons:

1. the education and training of medical personnel is a time consuming and costly affair. Medical personnel is highly educated and therefore highly specialized. Acquiring other skills is difficult, time consuming and signifies a waste of effort and money.
2. medical education and training is very costly, therefore educational planning and medical planning have to go hand in hand. A cynic might say that manpower planning for a reduction of the expected trend is less difficult than manpower planning for expansion. Expansion includes the setting up of new medical schools and faculties and at least the increase of the existing capacity. A reduction of the trend is possible by imposing a numerus clausus (student stop) in the existing faculties.

It is a possibility because on the basis of a budget the planning of the health sector has at least one hard and clear basic figure to work with, the OECD-study, on which the 1978 national seminar in the Netherlands was based, indicates that medical health care and medical education should be taken up together at the regional level, as was pointed out at that conference. (3)

1. It is possible to estimate costs of education and health care, because they are a joint production.
2. The planning of medical care and medical education has to include manpower planning.

Manpower planning then, is a necessity and a possibility in the health sector under the present circumstances. It tends to be a national affair carried out at the regional level. However, no nation, (not even the relatively big nations of Europe,) is an island. In the Common Market we have the free circulation of workers. In- and out-migration of all medical personnel was recognized by the European Commission as a logical consequence of this principle.

The Council accepted guidelines with regard to the mutual recognition of diploma's, certificates and other titles of the physicians, and other measures to facilitate the actual practice of the right to establish oneself within the member states and the freedom to perform services, in 1975. In 1977 it accepted guidelines with regard to the mutual recognition of diploma's and so on of nursing personnel. In the same year the European Commission decided to institute a committee of senior civil servants of national health of the member countries. This Committee has as its task to find and study difficulties that develop concerning the functioning of these guidelines, and to advise the Commissions concerning possible necessary changes in these guidelines.

In practice these guidelines have facilitated the migration of physicians and other medical personnel between the countries of the EEC. In The Netherlands since 1976 each year between 75 and 100 medical doctors and especially specialists establish themselves. In the other EEC-countries we find comparable figures. Although the freedom to establish oneself as a specialist or general practitioner is not yet complete in all the member-countries, the sum total of migrating medical doctors was about 1,000. Not a really important movement, but a development with potentialities for the future.

The development as we have seen it up to now is important enough to dedicate a discussion to the possible effects of the free circulation and free establishment on the measures to limit the number of students in medicine in the different countries. France embarked last year on a policy of limiting the number of students admitted to the medical study rather strongly from 14,000 in 1978 to 6,000 at present and not more than 5,000 in the near future.

Other countries follow different paths. It is clear that, given the freedom of circulation and of establishment the effectivenes of one governments' policy might be undermined by the policy of others.

What do we need?

I think that it is necessary to keep in mind that:

First: all the member states of the EEC have in different degrees the same kind of problems. In that sense there is a common necessity to find a solution.

Second: the field of manpower planning is characterized by uncertainties and unexpected difficulties. Moreover the fact that education of highly educated people takes time, plays an important role. In the meantime some data may be changing.

Third: medical education is so expensive and the financial problems of all governments are so pressing that it may be expected that the pressure for limitation of the number of students will increase. Governments may use different standards for the 'need' of medical personnel in the future, but it seems inevitable that a form of manpower planning enforced by legal measures will be introduced by one country after another.

Given the facts of Europe, national legislation will not be enough. Moreover without international regulations national legislation may loose its effectivity.

What form could international regulation take?

In the first place it is important that the field of manpower planning in health is not left to national studies only. The European Community should provide the framework for intensive discussion and common study of the existing and coming problems. This development in itself will lead to an approach towards a common view of the problems.

In the second place after careful study, covering the whole field of manpower in health, including physicians, specialists and nurses, the Community should develop European guidelines for national legislation in the field of manpower planning.

It would be unwise to expect that suddenly there will be only manpower planning at the European levels. More and more we become convinced that the actual mechanisms for manpower planning should be established within the nations at the regional level. But the working of the free movement principle will force us even against the built-in objections of national bureaucrats and politicians into the direction of international legislation.

Discussion

Kielty: commented that the speaker limited himself to the European theatre and wondered, in view of the lack of medical manpower elsewhere in the

world, whether European planning shouldn't take account of broader international needs.
Albeda: agreed.
Seiler: asked the speakers opinion on the 'normal' income level for a medical practitioner.
Albeda: discussed this from the Dutch viewpoint. He described how the Dutch authorities are trying to fix 'norm-incomes' by comparing the tasks of a doctor to a pre-existing function in public administration. The basic income of the doctor will then be based on that of the functionary, with additional emunerations to cover the costs of running a private practice. Thus the normative income of the doctor can be calculated. The Netherlands attempts to work within the framework of an international income policy to establish norms for incomes of all professions, including the medical. Further Albeda said 'This is not one of the most easy policies that we have to deal with, but I think it is really worthwile because in a time of depression, when you have the feeling that everybody has to do a step back, it is impossible to convince for instance the trade-unions, to make a step back if they don't have the feeling that at the same time, the government is studying the normative relationship that there should be between the income level of the different people in the labour market'.

References

1. In: Human Capital Formation and Manpower Development, R.A. Wijkstra Editor, New York 1971, p. 469.
2. Henry David, A perspective on manpower theory and conceptualization in 'Manpower for mental health', Franklin & Arnhoff e.a., Editors, Chicago 1969.
3. Cooperation of health care and education at regional level, OECD, Paris 1978.

Manpower Planning in Industrial Organizations and as a Necessity for Industrial Innovation

G.A. Wagner, M.A. Law

Mr chairman, ladies and gentlemen,

I must admit that it was at first with some hesitation that I agreed to speak at this symposium. I am an industrialist and by no means an expert in health manpower planning, and I realized that by accepting to speak to you today, you would expect me to shape my address in such a manner, that it would be useful for your deliberations. That would then force me to become more knowledgeable about your problems. Fortunately, in preparing this address I enjoyed the help of a much better informed colleague.

Health manpower planning is receiving considerable public attention in this country, particularly in recent years. As you know, also industry is wrestling these days with considerable manpower problems, and although over the years we may have accumulated more experience than you in this field, that does not make our problems any simpler. In what I am going to say, manpower planning in industry will be central, but in view of the fact that I cannot help holding certain views on your problems, I will digress from time to time into your area. In doing this I hope to provide you with the contrast you are looking for and it may perhaps give you some inspiration to find solution for your own problems.

I must emphasize right at the beginning that I do not believe you could just copy the way we approach our problems. On the other hand, certain notions we have developed will certainly be applicable to you as well and it is on those that I intend to concentrate.

Is a comparison between industry and the health sector meaningful?

Let us first consider the question of a comparison between the health sector and industry in some greater detail and ask ourselves whether such a comparison can be meaningful.

There is no doubt that the centripetal forces in industry are stronger, that within the framework of delegation of authority to the various units concerned, there is still a measure of central coordination and within a country even of central direction. In your world, manpower numbers are the result of a large number of individual decisions, with a minimum of central direction and guidance. Furthermore, for the majority of university graduates (and equivalent) employed in industry (such as engineers, chemists, physicists, economists, lawyers, accountants, etc.) there is a much greater diversity in their deployment than for health professionals. In fact many employees in industry will during their career digress considerably from their original field of study. I could name you examples of physicists and chemical engineers that now work as marketing men, of mechanical and electrical engineers that have become personnel managers, of erstwhile tanker officers that are now under training to become computer specialists. At first sight this might make the impression of being a wasteful practice, but in reality I think it is not. A tremendous enrichment of experience and a cross fertilization between disciplines will result from this practice. We believe people are flexible and we attach significance to their functional and geographical mobility, to their ability to adapt to different circumstances. Over the years we have developed the philosophy of 'growing our own timber'. We therefore rather see people specialize in greater depth, in a particular field of knowledge, whilst they are in our employment, than whilst they are at the university.The decisions by the organization and the individual as to who should specialize, when, where, on what and for how long are then taken on a fairly firm basis.

I clearly see here significant differences with the health sector: there large numbers of young people, very early in their life, are taking seemingly irrevocable decisions about their future, without personal experience and without much counselling and guidance. In your world, I believe, there is little of what we would call career planning and career counselling, by somebody who has a better overview of the prospects and a better overall picture, and who may then try to influence people to change direction. Moreover, medical practitioners are reputed for their individualism and one may wonder how much identification they have with the health system as a whole. Lead times can be very long and career lines are usually much shorter than in industry. In industry, if all is well, there is strong identification of employees with the company; they are part of that company and the company's goals are as important to achieve as their own personal goals. Do not be mistaken, the loyalty, dedication, 'sense of mission' if you like, of a research worker or of an engineer running a plant (to name a few), will be as great as that of a medical officer in say a hospital.

These are then indeed important differences from which, however, we can draw some useful conclusions:

1. Without advocating that there should be a unitary system, with central control and excessive limitation of the freedom of individuals, I believe that in 'health' more work could be done to make forecasts of developments in the job market, to guide students and to bring more flexibility in their career objectives. I will revert to this question later.

2. As regards future developments, I contend industry is subject to much greater uncertainty than 'health': companies are often at the mercy of the whims of consumers, of politicians, governments, suppliers of raw materials, of sudden variations in exchange rates and rates of interest, quite apart from the far from predictable market they serve. Although some of these factors apply to 'health' as well, in your world one should be able to find clear pointers from the demographic developments in a country as to the services that are needed in the future.

Let me elaborate.

Formal manpower planning systems in industry

There is the simple truth that if one aims to achieve a certain goal, one must prepare for it. And there is the equally simple truth, that if something has gone wrong, steps must be taken to remedy the situation. It would seem to me that manpower practices in industry mirror these two basic truths: we are not only concerned with expectations and plans for the future, but also with the inheritance of the past.

1. A classic example of the first category is a 'greenfield project' to build a plant, where one has to start from scratch. Demand has to be estimated, the size of the plant to be established, design work and construction has to be taken in hand, preparations have to be made for the recruitment, training and development of the staff that will have to run the plant.
2. An example of the second category is one, where things have gone wrong. There is, for instance, excess production capacity, plants must be closed, people become surplus to requirements. The original decision to build such production capacity was undoubtedly taken in good faith and nobody is to blame. We all know that these are difficult problems and that it may take some time before one is able to extricate oneself from a decision that has proved to be wrong.

Manpower planning in industry is usually a mixture of these two base types.

Many people join industry in the expectation of a lifelong career, but it is only rarely that industry can offer a career without major risks. Formal systems of manpower planning will usually improve the quality of decisions, but there is no guarantee that one will be right. There will always be unexpected developments, misjudgements, disappointments. Unpopular decisions need to be taken, and one should have the courage to take them early and with determination.

There was a time that many of us believed that forecasting, in essence, was not such a difficult task and that if only sufficient skill, time and energy was devoted to it, simple unique forecasts could be made of the most important factors determining our business. There was then some sensitivity analysis testing the consequences of a margin of error upwards and downwards. This type of forecasting was typical for the 50's and for the 60's. It has now become quite clear that this is no longer appropriate for the circumstances in which we will find ourselves in the 80's and the 90's. In the last 10–15 years Shell has pioneered in the development of scenarios, providing a backdrop of two to three different, but internally consistent futures, against which forecasts can be made, objectives set, strategies and operating programmes can be established. It would take me too far to go into great detail at this moment, and it is sufficient to say at this moment that this scenario approach is valid for all parts of the business, including manpower planning.

Having these scenarios as a starting point, as a common frame of reference, it is then up to us to decide what we will do with them. What are now our own expectations for the future, what will be the demand for our products, how will we be organized to serve our customers, what will be the effect of developments in technology and productivity on manpower levels? Having gone through a number of mental exercises, we then arrive at estimates of manpower needs a number of years ahead, where possible split by skill groups and with great attention to a harmonious age build-up so that proper succession in jobs over time is assured. This process enables us to establish recruitment levels, but also where in the course of time bottlenecks will occur and where therefore corrective measures will be needed. You will understand that in the time allotted to me, I cannot possibly do justice to how this system works in detail, and I can only draw the broad lines. Regular updates of manpower estimates are necessary, say every two years, to allow for new information, changes in plans, differences in assumptions.

Here again I would like to draw a contrast with 'health'. I have been informed that this type of projection into the future is often not made and that it is more common to let the capacity of educational institutes decide how many people will be educated for a particular profession. This is of course also true for other disciplines, but in your own case, in view of the relative inflexibility of deployment of people, it may have grave consequences. It is difficult to find a rationale for this approach and the mere fact that projections are difficult to make, is no excuse for not trying at all. I permit myself three suggestions at this moment in time, which would not only apply to your sector but to other sectors as well:

1. Elaborating on my earlier point, I believe that new generations of students, applying for places at universities and other educational institutes, should have access to estimates, produced by government or by an independent body, as to the job opportunities that can be expected when they have completed their studies. They should also have an opportunity to be counselled. It is hoped that this will set in motion

adaptation processes which will bring supply and demand closer together.

2. If there is surplus capacity at universities and educational institutes, such capacity should be brought into line with true needs in order to avoid wasting human and financial assets.
3. Finally, I believe that in a certain number of countries we can blame rigidities in the income structure to be the reason for a continuation of imbalances in the job market. If a particular skill is in over-supply, its income should drop, and if there is an under-supply, its income should increase. If we continue to pay high incomes in a sector where there is an over-supply, it will continue to attract people who hope that the general picture does not apply to them and that they can continue to enjoy the privileges of higher income as before.

Concern for productivity

When speaking about forecasts for longer term manpower needs in industry, I mentioned productivity as one of the determining factors. If we in Western Europe want to preserve our place amongst the leading industrial nations of the world, we need to be alive, not only to new opportunities and to innovation, but also to the need for maintaining a high level of productivity. In some cases this will lead to mechanisation and automation and therefore to replacement of human labour, in other cases it will mean economizing on overhead support staff. These developments cannot be artificially stopped for the sake of maintaining employment; companies that are not active in this area will soon find that they have become uncompetitive. An element of manpower planning is therefore the constant scrutiny of manning levels and the setting up of monitoring devices. I firmly believe that productivity criteria apply as much to the public sector as to the private sector and I have noted with great interest the tendency in a number of countries towards contracting our public services to private organizations, of course subject to strict rules. This is also known under the name 'privatisation of public services' – hospitals, public transport and other forms of public services could fall under this heading. The net outcome will usually be a reduction in manpower levels with the same level of service, of elimination of wasteful capital and revenue expenditure and hence lower costs. However, the need for productivity is so great that we should strive for it, irrespective of the possibilities of privatisation.

Supporting personnel systems

In our industry, decisions on manpower lie in the hands of line management. However, in carrying out this task, they have at their disposal personnel planning support systems. Many personnel planning specialists will come from the line themselves, so that they have an intimate knowledge of what is needed. Each major function in our organization will have its own personnel manager who has to see to it that decisions can be taken on the basis of adequate information. Careers are managed to the best of their ability, so that a more or less logical pattern emerges. You should not get the impression that we are overdirective in this field and that the company always knows best. In real life, there is much consultation and employees should of course agree to career moves that are proposed to them. There is much counselling, particularly when people need to be guided in a different direction than they had hoped for or which they would have expected. But if they are unwilling or uninterested, they would be both unhappy and unsuitable. We have an elaborate system of staff reporting, both on performance and on development and in addition there are regular staff discussions where career plans are discussed.

As so often, there is not one single description that fits the situation. In one part of the business, which we usually designate as downstream oil (refineries, supply and marketing organizations) there is contraction, restructuring and surplus manpower. Another example of the same kind is to be found in the necessary contraction of our tanker fleet. These processes of contraction can be painful and their implementation may often cover a period of several years. Then there is that part of our activities which finds itself in expansion, as for instance our exploration and production sector, our coal business or our manufacturing ventures overseas. Here, more people are needed, quite often with technical qualifications. We are recruiting for these needs and we also undertake a considerable training and re-training effort, often phased out in time so as to coincide with the accumulation of more experience on the job. It stands to reason that we try as often as possible to re-channel people from sectors that are in surplus, to sectors that are in deficit. This is not always easy and there are disappointments. You should therefore not get the impression that we have found the 'magic wand' and that we succeed in bringing this about quickly and without friction. However, some generalizations are possible. Older people usually pose greater problems than younger people; further development potential is usually favourable for redeployment. People in their thirties are normally retrainable, redeployabele. If the problem is identified early enough, sensible solutions can usually be found.

Knowing that also in 'health' there are in certain countries manpower surplusses, I hope that these observations will have some relevance for your own situation.

Innovation

Let us now look to the future, to manpower planning as a necessity for industrial innovation. It should be clear that innovation in industry in the broadest sense is not just a matter of formal effort, but is even more the outcome of the organizational climate. Is the organization responsive to new developments in society, do we really encourage those qualities in people, like 'entrepeneurship', commercial sense, inventiveness, social awareness that will lead to industrial success? We believe our manpower planning practices, which pay so much attention to the development of the individual, do indeed contribute to this cause. The generating of new ideas has indeed to be encouraged, but it should be tempered by a certain realism, by the knowledge that certain ideas will prove to be not viable. We must admit that the process of innovation can be wasteful and that a lot of ideas are pursued that are not worth pursuing. If we succeed in developing sensible people, oriented towards results and not towards innovation for its own sake, we will have discharged our responsibilities in the best possible manner.

We do indeed recruit and develop people with an eye on developments, (technical, social and commercial,) which we expect in the late 80's and 90's. It is a matter of careful selection of our staff that are most suitable for these tasks, of seeding the required expertise into the organization, but also of maintaining a constant inflow of young people, so that we keep abreast of what society expects and dictates.

Summary

My main message can be summed up as follows:

1. Despite differences, the health sector would indeed benefit from having a look at manpower planning practices in industry.
2. As in business, the health sector should develop a general frame of reference, that cristallizes expectations of future developments and against which individual decisions can be put.
3. In the light of the foregoing there should be more information given to students as to job opportunities; there should be more counselling and the market mechanism should be allowed to bring about realistic differentiations in pay levels.
4. It is vital that the health sector gets a clear view of its own productivity, contracting out of some public services to private organizations could provide a useful cross-check.
5. A long term view is a necessary backdrop for short term decisions; we should be recruiting and developing now the young people that will be concerned with the 'technologies' of the 90's.

Discussion

Greep: disagreed with the analogy between health care and consumer-product relationships at least relative to how clinicians define the needs of their (sick) patients.
Wagner: said that although he drew on industrial analogies that are not directly comparable to the health care scene, however some situations are similar, for instance the responsibility of the specialist towards younger doctors.
Milton: on re-education; in citing the current trend in Sweden to favour older people in admission to re-education programmes asked whether the speaker thought that there is an optimum age for beginning re-education.
Wagner: highly specialized professionals should be selected before the age of 35. If older it must be considered an 'emergency' measure which may or may not work out.

A Conceptual Framework for Health Manpower Planning

Dev. K. Ray, M.D., Ph.D.

Introduction

The World Health Organization has set itself the target of achieving health for all by the year 2000, that is, to maintain all the people of the world at a sufficiently positive level of health so that they can lead economically and socially productive lives. One of the contributions to positive health is health care, which is usually personal care. Health care demands the intervention of individuals - whether health workers of family members - for the prevention and treatment of diseases.

Health services, which provide the bulk of health care - at least curative care - are thus particularly labour-intensive; much of the money required to run health services is allocated to salaries of personnel. The proportion of total cost devoted to salaries in order to run the health services can be as high as 60% to 70%. It is, therefore, necessary to use manpower wisely, especially when lack of trained manpower is often the stumbling block in the delivery of health care to all.

Manpower planning aims to ensure that the required numbers of appropriate personnel are available at the proper time and in the right place to staff the health services. However, human resources have some characteristics which set them apart from other resources such as facilities, equipment and money. For example,

- the behaviour patterns and skills of individuals differ and consequently they cannot easily be substituted one for another;
- individuals cannot be stored for future use, nor discarded at will;
- health personnel may leave the services when they wish;
- trained manpower cannot be produced at short notice; for professional workers up to a decade may elapse between the decision to train and the availability of such workers;
- performance of individuals depends to a large extent om motivation, conditions of service, career opportunities, etc.

All these characteristics make the task of planning for manpower difficult and yet essential for the proper delivery of health care.

New directions in health manpower development

The WHO/UNICEF International Conference on Primary Health Care, held in Alma Ata, declared that primary health care would be the cornerstone of a strategy to attain health for all by the year 2000. This calls for a tremendous reorientation of priorities, resources and attitudes. The conference recommended that primary health care be delivered through 'teams composed of community health workers, other developmental workers, intermediate personnel, nurses, midwives, physicians and, where applicable, traditional practitioners and traditional birth attendants'. In addition, it recommended 'that health workers, especially physicians and nurses, should be socially and technically trained and motivated to serve the community'. In order to attain the goal of health for all by the year 2000, not only strategies for implementing primary health care to be developed carefully, but also plans for health manpower development have to be established which will lead to adequate human resources to deliver the appropriate health care. It is in the planning and implementation stages that countries often fall short of the objectives.

The World Health Organization recognized the need for planning as an integral part of the total health manpower planning in its Sixth General Programme of Work (1978-1983) (1) prepared in 1976. Its Seventh General Programme of Work (1984-1989) (2), to be discussed by the World Health Assembly in May of this year, sets out the objective of its health manpower development programme as 'to promote, and cooperate with countries in planning for, training and deploying the number and types of personnel they require and can afford; and to help ensure that such personnel are socially responsible and possess appropriate technical, scientific and management competences, so as to develop and maintain comprehensive national health systems based on primary health care for the attainment of health for all by the year 2000'.

The three main elements of the health manpower development process are planning, production and management of health manpower (figure 1). The term 'production' is used for convenience to denote the training and continuing education of health manpower. In practice, in many countries all these elements do not exist. Even where they do exist there is often a lack of coordination between the elements. Health manpower plans, where they exist, are drawn up independently by the training institutions. Yet health manpower production is the task of these training institutions; they define the numbers to be trained and the training curricula - often independently of the service needs. In addition, there are significant problems in health manpower management - there is seldom any monitoring and feedback to check whether the health workers are being properly utilized, whether they are able to cope with the tasks for which they were trained, and what the needs are for updating their competence and job satisfaction,

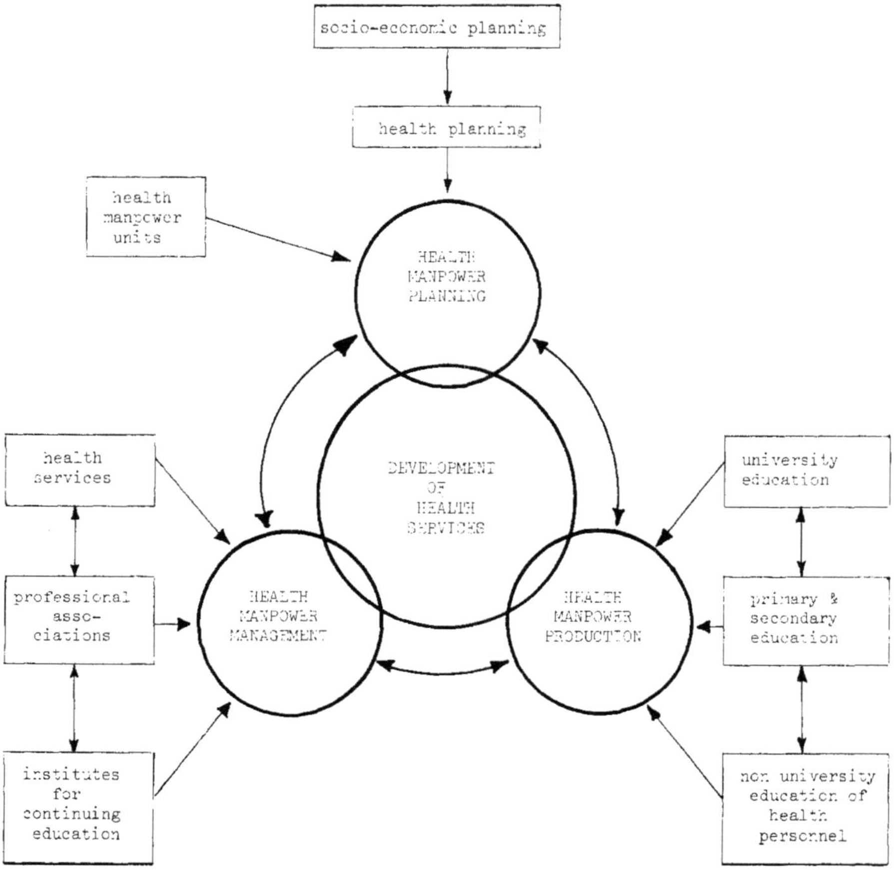

National bodies involved: ministry of Health (or equivalent), ministry of Social Welfare (or equivalent), ministry of Education (or equivalent), ministry of Socio-Economic Development (or equivalent), ministry of Planning (or equivalent), ministry of Labour (or equivalent), National Research Institutes, etc.

Figure 1 Institutional interrelationship between Health Service and Manpower Development (HSMD) and some of the national bodies involved (3)

as well as life and working conditions. Thus, health manpower development has elements which act quite independently and, so far, do not support one another effectively.

Role of health manpower planning

One of the tasks of strengthening health manpower development is not only to institute the three elements mentioned earlier, but to ensure their coordination. If integrated development of health manpower is to be consonant with health service needs, health manpower planning must play an indispensable role. It would be instrumental in ensuring that realistic plans are drawn up, that the plans are implemented, and that the three elements are coordinated during the processes of implementation. The manner and degree of such coordination will, of course, vary from country to country.

Manpower planners have, so far, considered their tasks to be limited to projecting future requirements and supply of manpower and to highlighting interventions to rectify the imbalances. The central element in the whole process has been the forecasting of future manpower requirements, and progressively more and more sophisticiated tools have been used for this purpose. In spite of much work in this area, many manpower forecasting efforts have proved to be less than successful. The reasons for these failures are manifold; among them is the obsession of planners with numbers. Very little attention has been paid to the analysis of manpower policies and the relevance of training to service needs. This has led to an uneconomic use of manpower when highly.qualified personnel have been delivering care which lies within the competence of less qualified personnel. The lack of a clear definition of functions, and an absence of basing training curricula on these functions, have led to deficiencies in the quality of health care provided and to maldistribution of health resources within countries.

Furthermore, national health planning has paid little attention to health manpower planning. Usually requirements for health manpower are based on health plans that contain only statements of how many of what categories of manpower would be needed for the implementation of the plans. This is only the first step in the manpower planning process as it ignores the long-term implications of such planning, as well as the orientation of the educational processes and the need to satisfy the manpower requirements of services. Relatively little attention is paid to the building of training institutions, the training of teachers, the role continuing education, and the career prospects of the health workers. There have been many consequences of such inadequate planning, where training institutions have been expanded at a rapid rate. A large number of health workers could then not be absorbed by the health services and their training was irrelevant to the needs of the health services.

Such experiences with health planning and health manpower planning led to the conclusion that manpower planning should be more concerned with the actual decision-making process and implementation of decisions than with the manipulation of numbers in forecasting demand and supply. Health manpower planning is recognized as being more political and social than mathematical. Planning efforts are unlikely to be effective if due account is not taken of the social, economic and the political milieu in which they take place.

In addition, the previous ad hoc efforts of WHO to organize numerous seminars and symposia, although useful, gradually came to be seen as not fully effective. The seminars, not being followed by an actual health manpower planning exercise, remained somewhat academic; the subject matter was presented piecemeal instead of in the sequence that would be used by an actual manpower planner. The seminars also tended to be organized at the inter-country level, with the result that there were seldom enough nationals trained from the same country to make an impact on their country's planning capabilities. Moreover, the provision of consultants to draw up the actual manpower plans appeared increasingly to be an outmodel form of support: this was technical assistance, with its notion of donor aid to a recipient, rather than technical cooperation between partners, the new mode which the Organization was striving to adopt. Out of this conviction of the need for a new approach grew the first effort to develop a set of Guidelines for Health Manpower Planning (4) that would complement a previous WHO publication on the subject (5) and that could serve as a course book as well as an actual planning tool. Used at the national level, it could facilitate the training of a 'critical mass' of manpower planners who could then take over the task of producing a manpower plan – making a consultant unnecessary.

Workshop plus planning: learning by doing

The current approach is to organize national training courses (given in the form of a workshop or seminar) after which the newly trained nationals formulate their own health manpower plan for the country. This immediate application of the trainees' newly acquired knowledge strengthens their motivation to learn, as well as resulting in a manpower plan of practicial use to their country. In keeping with the technical cooperation approach, the role of external consultants during the workshop is limited to that of catalysts. This is also true of their role during the formulation of the national manpower plan, if they participate at all in this phase; the formulation process is sometimes conducted entirely by nationals.

The Guidelines are intended for administrators and educators concerned with initiating, directing, or conducting planning efforts, or with training others in health manpower planning. The trainees may be drawn from national, regional, or local settings, but if the second phase – the formulation of a health manpower plan – has to be fruitful, the participants must occupy posts at the decision-making level.

The Guidelines are a set of ten procedural steps for planning health manpower, developed after considerable testing in a variety of country workshops. The actual organization and conduct of workshops and formulation efforts necessarily vary from country to country, just as the procedural steps outlined in the guidelines need adaptation in each instance to the local situation. But the basic principle involved seems to be sound. The combined workshop and formulation approach results in a cadre of trained manpower planners and a health manpower plan that is truly own. The external consultants who might have catalyzed the process may not even be in agreement with the final plan. In any event they are soon forgotten: they have made themselves redundant through technical cooperation.

Ten Steps to Health Manpower Planning

Health manpower planning and health planning are processes which attempt to identify ways to achieve certain targets within the limits of available resources and to resolve or prevent mismatches between the requirements and availability of manpower. Notwithstanding the cyclical nature of manpower planning, a set of steps are proposed in figure 2 to be followed in health manpower planning. These steps are presented in a sequence, but certain adjustments may be needed for an actual planning activity. Some steps may be omitted from the proposed sequence and it may be necessary to move repeatedly between other steps.

Health manpower planning begins when a government or organization decides to undertake it. When such a decision is made, areas of concern and the expected outcome must be specified. A group of health manpower planners should include representatives of health service organizations, health manpower development institutions, professional bodies and other interested groups. Such a group should be fully aware of the country's political orientation and the long-term social and development priorities.

Once such a group is formed, information about health services and manpower development must first be collected and presented. Often such data are already available but sometimes a manpower situation report may have to be produced based on raw information obtained from data sources. Subsequently, the future supply of manpower has to be estimated on the availability of current manpower, the rates of leaving and future additions to the staff. Future manpower requirements may be estimated in terms of quality, quantity, productivity and distribution of staff, using a variety of different approaches:

1. The health needs approach based on expert opinion about the amount and nature of health services needed to attain and preserve the health of populations;
2. The service targets approach which identifies targets for the provision of various kinds of health services based on diverse criteria of needs and feasibility;
3. The health demands approach estimating the effective economic demand for services as a function of income, price, accessibility, etc., and

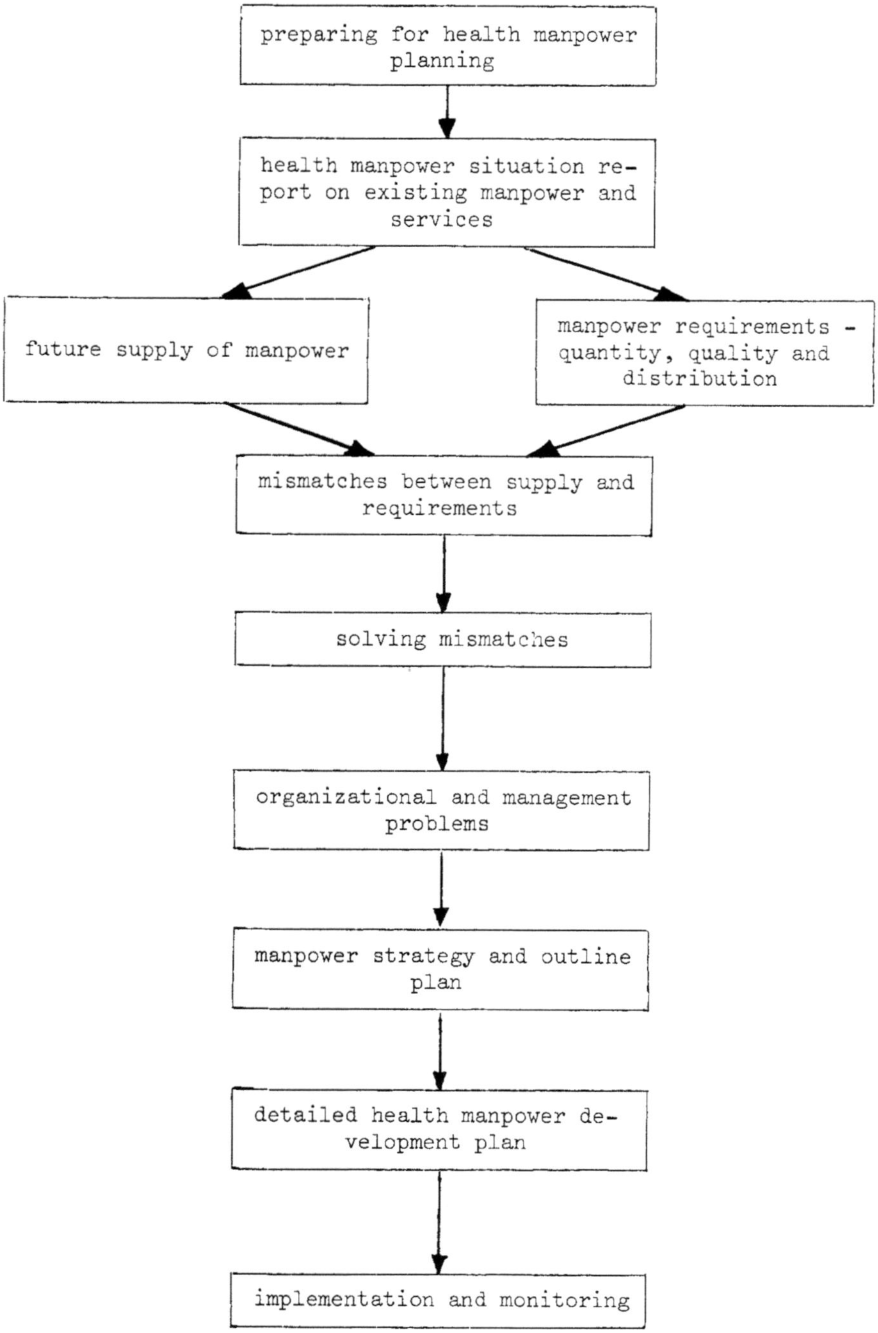

Figure 2 Procedural steps in Health Manpower Planning

4. Manpower population ratios using desirable or empirical normative ratios.

In reality a combination of these approaches may be used.

The future supply of manpower and manpower requirements can now be compared which will reveal mismatches. There may be too few or too many of various categories of staff; needed skills may be lacking; productivity may be low; the costs may be too high and there may be a geographical maldistribution of staff. Once the problems have been identified and broadly clarified, the manpower planning group should list all major alternative solutions to them. In selecting between solutions it is normal to first concentrate on those which are of a long-term nature and which can be absorbed gradually within the projected availability of resources. The effects of these actions may not be visible for a long time. Subsequently, many of the resource-based solutions will have to be examined to satisfy certain short-term commitments requiring radical changes in policy or action. Each such solution must then be scrutinized to ensure that it is feasible. Constraints in the situation may make some solutions impossible to achieve while other solutions may simply face obstacles that can be circumvented.

The different organizational and management implications can be classified in five broad categories:

1. Coordination between health service development and manpower development.
2. Educational planning to ensure relevance of training to the needs of service.
3. Effective management of manpower.
4. Career development prospects, and
5. Continuing education to support career development and maintain and supplement the skills of manpower.

At this stage an outline plan could be developed and discussed by different interested parties so that policy guidance can be obtained before finalizing the detailed plan. The detailed plan should include schedule of activities, the budgetary requirements and milestones to monitor the progress of implementation of the plan.

Manpower planning is not finished when the final plan is produced. There must be continued involvement of the planner in the plan's implementation, both in order to interact with those responsible for actions as well as to enable future modifications of the plans. If the full potential of the planning process has to be realized, and the plan used as an effective tool of management, decisionmakers must not just accept plan changes but rather expect them.

Conclusion

The global strategy for achieving health for all by the year 2000 calls for planning health manpower in specific response to the needs of the health system and for reviewing training programmes in the light of projections of the number, types, and quality of health workers required. Health manpower planning is an integral part of the total managerial process and should be meshed with health planning, programming, budgeting, and evaluation. Initially, however, given the special complexities of planning for this particular resource, countries may need to develop health manpower planning separately, in parallel with the other managerial processes, until its full integration becomes possible.

Discussion

Leer: drew the attention of the speakers to the fact that the medical 'company' employs not only clinicians but also non-clinicians whose job-needs are equally important.
Brearley Jr: asked the speaker why he thought that efforts towards national manpower planning seem more succesfull than towards international manpower planning.
Ray: it is more succesfull to tackle a specific problem of one particular group in a particular region; this could be sub-national, national or, as in the case of for instance migration, international.

References

1. WHO Official Records, no. 233, 1976, p. 102.
2. WHO, Executive Board document, EB69/4, 1981, p. 62.
3. Fülöp, T., New Approaches to a permanent problem: the integrated development of health services and health manpower, *WHO Chronicle, 30* (11). 1976.
4. Hornby, P., Ray, D.K., Shipp. P.J. and Hall T.L. *Guidelines for Health Manpower Planning*, World Health Organization, Geneva, 1980.
5. Hall, T.L. & Majia, A., *Health Manpower Planning: principles, methods and issues*, World Health Organization, Geneva, 1980.

Relationship of Health Workers Training for Manpower Planning

Fr.C.A. Jaspers, M.D.

Introduction

After the lectures stressing the growing importance of manpower planning by mr Albeda and mr Wagner, dr Ray has set up a conceptual framework for Health Manpower Planning.

Today, it is my task to elaborate the relationship of health care and the training of health workers. In the case of The Netherlands, this is not a new issue. Already in 1978 a national seminar was organized by the Dutch ministries of Education and Sciences, and of Health and Environmental Protection in collaboration with the Organization for Economic Cooperation and Development (OECD). At this seminar on 'Cooperation of Health Care and Education at the Regional Level' the participants discussed extensively the problem of integrated planning of health services, the educational system and of the required manpower. In the same sense as at our symposium today, one of the aims was to learn from the experiences in other European countries, where the same problems prevail or have been overcome, and to see whether general guidelines for the process of health manpower development and planning are emerging. In this sense today's symposium is a follow-up of the national seminar of 1978. (1)

The planning of manpower of health care, and especially of physicians, is becoming more and more important as a policy-making instrument. Integrated health planning is necessary for a health policy adapted to social, economic and political developments. If one goes back in history, one can see, that this point of view has become a common opinion. However, in the case of The Netherlands, very little of this knowledge is translated in health care and educational policies. In 1968, at the end of the 'Working Symposium on Longe-Range Forecasting and Planning', the participants of this OECD-symposium stated, that 'social institutions face growing difficulties as a result of an ever increasing complexity, which arises directly and indirectly from the development and assimilation of technology. Many of the most serious conflicts facing mankind result from the interaction of social, economic, technological, political and psychological forces and can no longer be solved by fractional approaches from individual disciplines'. (2) In 1975, an OECD-Expert Committee made six proposals for action, of which two dealed with the planning of the health care and education systems, and this especially at the regional level. (3)

In The Netherlands this concept of regionalization and of integrated planning at this level, has not been established: cooperation between the health care system and the educational system is rudimentary at the national level and is completely absent at the regional or provincial level. Also there exist different and sometimes conflicting concepts about what health care should be. Sometimes one gets the impression that the financers of health care (i.e. the sickfunds and the insurance companies) are the main policy-makers. Government policy then becomes subsidary to the results of the negotiations between the medical profession and the insurance companies. We may hope that the conclusions and recommendations of today's symposium may result in changes and in new objectives for policy in a more extensive way than this has happened with those of the national seminar of 1978. In this lecture we will deal with the interrelationships between the health care system and the training system of health care workers, and especially of medical doctors. The following scheme shows the part of the health manpower process, we will discuss (figure 1).

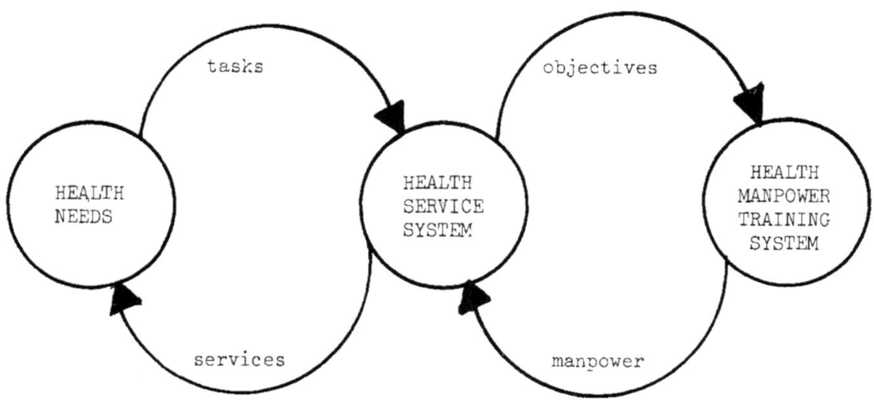

Figure 1 Approach of the health manpower planning process (after Van den Bussche and Reerink) (18)

The analysis of the interrelationships of health needs, health service system and health manpower training system, relates only to the industrialized countries, and especially the Western-European countries. We will focus on the interrelationships of the health service system and the health manpower training system. The Dutch situation will be used as an example, because we are most familiar with it. We are dealing with an existing system of health services and an existing health manpower training system; we will pay attention in the first place to the shifts in the interrelationships of these two systems. The intertwining of the health care system with the health manpower training system makes it impossible to talk about the first without taking the latter into account. The interrelationships are reflected in figure 1 by the two arrows: objectives and manpower. These arrows represent the relationship between the one system and the other.

Developments in health care since World War-II

Several developments in health care and educational systems, which are important to us today took place in industrialized countries during the last decades: (4)

- an enormous scaling up, mostly in the so-called intra-mural sector, as a consequence of an demand of the population for health care (and education);
- an exponential rising of costs and the limitations of the economic possibilities;
- the call for external democracy ('explosion of human expectations');
- the increasing speed by which advances become obsolescent ('explosion of medical technology') and the slow reaction of the educational system to this turnover;
- the inertia of the health care system and its ineffectiviness.

All this led to a health policy of 'distributive' or 'allocative' health care administration. The intervention from the central administration – especially of governments – was limited: the knowledge of which processes were going on in the health sector was limited. Mostly the policy was fragmented and restricted to quantitative solutions of acutely raised problems (e.g. the threatening deficit of physicians). In time this led to 'instant-policymaking'.

In the post-world-war-development, one can differentiate four periods in health care policy:

1. Period of rebuilding: everyone helped to restore the destroyed health care and educational system;
2. Period of deficits of qualified manpower: qualified personnel is indispensable for highly industrialized countries, like those of Western-Europe. One tried to manage these problems with methods lent from the economical sciences; these methods were mainly quantitative methods of planning, restricted to physical and financial services. It was in essence 'crisis-management';
3. Period of stormy and uncontrolled expansion of services, manpower, finances and technology;
4. Period of renewal: gradually it became clear, that quantitative planning (this means: changes in size, pure and simple) can only appear to its full advantage if it is completed with qualitative planning (this means:

changes of any kind other than a change in size alone).
The policy-makers wanted also to fulfil the qualitative needs and demands from the society; it was no longer possible to suffice the society with higher budgets, and more and more beautiful buildings. The structure and the contents of the health care system came in the picture. This last period, started in the middle of the 70's, led to an explosion of official reports, seminars, etc. For example in The Netherlands, the so-called 'Structuur-nota' (1974) of the State Secretary Health, which represented a definite point of new-thinking in health care policy, and has led to a renewal of legislation. At this moment health planning and health manpower planning is considered as a process of continuous feedback, a 'rolling reform'.

On the other side we are confronted with a very difficult paradox: 'The particular situation, or systems state, in which we find ourselves today, is characterized by the necessity for planning on the one hand, and by the reluctance of the system to accept planning on the other'. (2) Perhaps the reason of this paradox is the efforts of planning on a too high level: one can solve this problem in the field of health sector by planning on the regional level and by means of budget-financing and budget-control. Because health manpower planning at the moment is taking place only at the national level in industrialized countries, and in a much lesser extent at the regional level, one cannot be surprised by this reluctance to planning; especially in those countries where medical doctors are working on a basis of fee-for-service-payment, as for instance in The Netherlands.

Dealing in the next part of this lecture in more detail with the interrelationships between the health care system and the manpower productive system, we have to bear in mind, that this planning has to be:

- an integrated process of planning;
- both a qualitative and quantitative process of planning;
- directed on the short, the middle and the long-term range;
- concentrated on changes and shifts within the health care system and in relation with the health manpower productive system.

In democratically governed countries health planning must be a process supporting decision-making by the elected and responsible institutions (e.g. the parliament). The results of the planning have to be subsidiary to the policy.

By this reason one has to avoid the 'technocratic model' of health (manpower) planning, in which science and planning dominate the decision-makers.

In the United Kingdom and the United States of America, the 'Committee System' is often used as a method of planning. In these committees science and administration are brought together. The committees are asked to make scientifically performed analyses and to generate political and administrative recommendations in solving the social problems. Excellent examples of this method were/are:

- Report of the Committee of Inquiry into the Regulation of the Medical Profession (Chairman: dr A.W. Merrison, F.R.S. (5)
- Report of the Interdepartmental Committee on Medical Schools (Chairman: Sir William Goodenough) (6)
- Report of the Royal Commission on Medical Education (Chairman: The Rt. Hon. The Lord Todd, D.SC., F.R.S.) (7)
- Report of the Graduate Medical Education National Advisory Committee (Chairman: Alvin R. Tarlov, M.D.) (8)

In The Netherlands this system of planning is not used so extensily; we know a more rudimentary committee-system, in which more superficial reports are made, which are not often followed by or translated in administrative actions.

The objectives of the health service system to the health manpower training system

Although we are not dealing with an ideal health care system in the Western-European countries, a kind of general theory of health care has recently been developed. (1, 2 and 3) The impetus was given by the unmanageable costs of the health care system in the western highly industrialized countries.

The health care system of western countries is so large and complex, that it consumes 8% to 10% of the Gross National Product (GNP), and employs 5% to 6% of the labour force. Personnel salaries account for 60% to 80% of the costs of health care today. In figure 2 we can see the distribution of labour in the Dutch Health Service, and its division in two subsystems.

Of the total labour force 4/5 is working in the intramural setting, the system that admits the somatical sick and mentally ill people for diagnosis,

	1975	1980	1985
total personnel	237,794	277,660	326,523
intramural	85.3%	84.3%	82.7%
extramural	9.0%	10.2%	11.5%
other	5.7%	5.5%	5.8%

Figure 2 Labour in the Dutch Health Service and its distribution; source: Financial Survey, 1982 (9)

treatment and care. The extramural setting, elsewhere called 'primary health care', functions in for example, The Netherlands and the United Kingdom, as the entrance to the entire health care system. Its major problem in industrialized countries is the medicalization of social problems. (10)

The hospital sector absorbs in western countries generally 2/3 of the equipment and resources of the entire system (figure 3).

	1975	1980	1985
total costs	17,038	27,774	43,753
intramural	64.2%	65.1%	59.5%
extramural	16.0%	16.1%	16.4%
general preventive care	2.5%	2.7%	2.8%
other	17 3%	16 1%	21 3%

Figure 3 Costs of the Dutch Health Service in millions of guilders and the distribution of the expenditure; source: Financial Survey, 1982 (9)

Therefore it is understandable that most of the attention in regard with (medical) manpower planning is directed to the hospital care system. Since 60% to 80% of the costs go to salaries manpower planning is one of the major instruments in cost containment in the health care system (figure 4).

	in millions of guilders	distribution of total expenditure
salaries, social contributions and other personnel costs	5,382	68.5%
food	175	2.2%
drugs, dressings, etc.	792	10.1%
depreciation	372	4.7%
interest	448	5.7%
sundry costs	689	8.8%
total	7,858	100.0%

Figure 4 Expenditure of Dutch hospitals and type of expenditure in 1978; source: CBS, 1980 (11)

The final aim for the total health care system is to make available to the entire population what can be offered economically. Whatever we do, it must be efficient and efficacious, in the sense of availability, accessibility and continuity. Because 80% to 90% of all patients can be treated in the primary care situation, it is a mistake, that the percentage spent on primary care will not increase in relation to the decrease of the intramural sector (figure 3 and ref. 2).

This all is stressing the growing importance of planning health services and the required manpower. The first recommendation of an OECD-Expert Committee, accepted by the OECD-Council, stated: 'clearly expressed national health policies should be developed, preferably by permanently-established planning mechanisms in which providers and consumers of health care play a participatory role'. (3) Planning of the required manpower is secondary to the planning of health, but the crucial question remains: what are the objectives of a satisfactory health care system in regard to the health manpower training system?

For an industrialized country, it is difficult to answer the 'needs and demands'. Using these words we apply a normative terminology. Is the objective to prolong life expectancy, to prevent illness, or to improve quality of living? Mostly the two key-issues of the manpower planning models are: (13)

- the physician manpower requirements, which are related to the incidence and prevalence or epidemiology of diseases;
- the evaluation process of the needs and demands, which is adapted to the manpower requirements, based upon several models and processes.

This view is restricted to quantitative estimates, but it should also include estimates on (13 and 14): changes in medical technology, treatment modalities, patient preferences, careseeking behaviour, provision of care, expected prevalence of diseases in regard to prevention and administration services, government policy at both legislative and executive levels, physician workloads, tasks and roles of paramedical workers, non-patient care activities as teaching and research, and questions about the entire educational continuum. One of the most recent efforts to do this was the exhaustive study - which has tried to encompass all these factors (included the estimate of supply and requirements) - of GMENAC in the USA. (8) This study tries to formulate the above mentioned objectives of the health care system to the manpower training system.

The Tools for Health Manpower Planning

In 1978, when the health care system in The Netherlands consumed 26 thousand million guilders (8,6% of GNP), the population also consumed

8,6 thousand million guilders (2,8% of GNP) for tobacco, soft drinks and alcoholic beverages; in the same year the educational system consumed 6,8% of GNP. (15) This observation raises questions about whether a society's legislation for health care should cover everything everybody desires and also whether it should leave options open for separate insurance coverage which enables people to choose between whiskey, tobacco and a coronary by-pass operation. This observation means also that governments have to make the choice, otherwise the development of the social (health care) system will be an intrinsic one; for example, the medical profession will regulate the development of the health care system. In the western countries we have arrived at the point, that we have to make the choice, because otherwise we will not evolve middle and long-term policies, which provide in a timely fashion an educational system which can perform its tasks satisfactorily and which keeps open the possibility of new scientific developments in health care through cost-containment of the existing facilities.

The tools to control these intrinsic autonomous processes are: regionalization of health services, national budget-control of the health care system, strictly balancing the supply and requirements of physicians and non-physicians, medical audit with feedback, education in cost of services, education in ordering protocols of clinical diagnosis and treatment, restrictions and rationing, positive/negative incentives, in medical audit with feedback of physicians (over-)ordering and perhaps banishing of the fee-for-service-payment. Yet each requires considerable effort to implement. (16)

The Dawson Report (1922) and the Goodenough Report (1944) (6) stated firstly the importance of the regionalization of health services. The already mentioned OECD-Expert Committee (3) put it forward in its recommendations: 'National health care policies should foster conjoint education/health care action at the regional level, and institutions at that level should establish mechanisms to implement such actions'.

The definitions of a region are based upon a 'complete set' of health care facilities together with all related teaching facilities, including an universitary (hospital). This last institution should be the center and top-service of a region, an item which we find not in the Dutch discussions about regionalization. For the western highly industrialized countries the size for each region is about one to two million people. Such a region will generate, by epidemiological studies and by research on the demands of the population and the professions, the requirements for physicians and paramedical workers. The estimate of the number of workers then has to be based upon the acceptable workload of each individual (in full-time and part-time functions). The fee-for-service-payment or the capitation-payment models of functioning of doctors are not reconcilable with this health care (manpower) planning model. One of the tools in this planning is like that of the

United Kingdom and many other countries, the system of 'house staffing', comprising housemen, junior and senior registrars, consultants, etc. House staffing will generate: changing of the payment system, acceptable workloads for physicians, planning facilities for the primary health care, adapted educational systems for physicians (region-centered), planning of health care facilities, specialities and hospital functions, and at least possibilities for (individual) career planning.

Relationship of Health Care and Health Care Workers Training for Manpower Planning.

The basic setting for productive cooperation between the health care system and the educational system and the basis for manpower planning, quality improvement and for cost-containment is theoretically defined. Intense cooperation is required between two large and complex systems, and this is only possible if three main conditions are fulfilled: adequate legislation, accountability and compliance. Legislation is necessary because this follows from national objectives and should provide the framework for control and for responsibilities, also in the financial sphere. Accountability is concerned with quality control. Workers-compliance is an essential condition. (15)

The main objective of the (needed) national legislation is: how to guarantee the best medical undergraduate, postgraduate and continuing education, in order to get the most efficient and efficacious health services for the population. This legislation should indicate the responsibilities and the financing of the educational system. A medical teaching institution can only function well when it is at least a fully-fledged partner in the control of the facilities or institutions of health care, which it needs for teaching. This is true for the entire medical educational continuum and not just the university hospitals.

The two service systems for education and for health care have much in common. Simplified the rough common characteristics of the educational and the health care system are:

- size is determined by level of wealth of a country;
- operate on principles of 'needs and demands';
- activities are mainly individual efforts;
- budget is 60% to 70% determined by salaries;
- stratification in primary, secondary, tertiary education or health facilities;
- quality control is difficult.

Both systems are linked through an extension of the meaning given to 'human rights' and are linked by the process of manpower planning, i.e. the production of qualified requirements of manpower. At the national level, this means:

- to the health care system: creating legislative and financial conditions for providing primary and secondary care for the entire population, and creating environmental health services;
- to the educational system: legislation, which guarantees facilities, teaching resources and financing for the entire educational system of physicians and non-physicians;
- to the two systems: development of a flexible system for health manpower planning at the regional and national level, and coordination of the legislation for the two systems.

Division of Labour between Physicians and Non-Physicians

It is obvious that - in the perspective of the projected oversupply of physicians - the requirements for non-physician health care providers (the paramedical workers) should be integrated into physician manpower planning.

Many non-physicians make positive contributions to the health care system. Mostly they are working under the supervision of physicians, not practicing independently.

They can enhance patient access to services, decrease costs and provide a broader range of services. In figure 5 the numbers of physicians and paramedical workers in the Netherlands are shown. The personnel of nursing homes and psychiatric institutions are excluded.

An inverse relationship exists between the number of physicians needed and the number of paramedical workers needed to provide a fixed number

	1975	1980	1985
medical specialists	4,949	6,065	7,350
general practitioners	4,809	5,468	7,000
dentists	3,930	5,087	6,250
district-nurses	4,074	4,857	?
maternities nurses	3,380	3,898	?
physiotherapists	3,000	5,500	8,600
nursing personnel in hospitals	54,750	58,150	?
medical, paramedical and auxiliary personnel in hospitals	21,300	27,754	?
general personnel in hospitals	40,920	44,360	?

Figure 5 Number of physicians and paramedical workers in the primary health care and hospital care in The Netherlands; source: Financial Survey, 1982 (9)

of medical services. In regard to manpower planning all paramedical workers should also be considered. Much more extensive study should be done in regard to the interrelationships of the tasks and functions of physicians and non-physicians. This research should include topics, such as (8 and 17):

- the effect of a physician excess on non-physician utilization;
- the relative costs and expenditures of using non- physicians instead of physicians for selected medical care services;
- the limits and reasons of consumer preference for and acceptance of paramedical workers;
- the problems of delegation and adequate supervision.

From all this, it follows that manpower planning for the health care system cannot be carried out by the medical profession alone, but is a responsibility of local, regional and national governments. Even on those levels the obstacles are great, of which historical background, expectations of the population and of the personnel interests of the health care professions are only a few. But without manpower planning on a national basis and the ensuing demands on the educational system, it is impossible to achieve optimal health care systems.

Acknowledgement

My sincere thanks go to professor A. Querido, M.D. (University of Leyden) and to professor S.A. Duursma, M.D. (University of Utrecht) for their stimulating discussions, helpful suggestions, and their reading of the manuscript.

Discussion

McNally: emphasized that what health care is going to be able to provide is decided by politicians and financial experts. Furthermore he suggested that the system of 'house staffing' may give junior doctors a better chance to choose an appropriate future specialization but also leads to a surplus of (qualified) juniors for the few specialist jobs. He also suggested that if 'fee-for-service' is abolished, the specialists salary is more easily defined and can become a *political* 'hot potato'.
Vissers: the speaker emphasized the necessity of relating the output of medical schools to the staffing needs of the health service. I ask the speaker's view as to who should control medical education, the ministry of Health or the ministry of Science and Education?
Jaspers: both: there should be close cooperation between those ministries.

Vissers: asked for a definition of the needs of health care, and from which point of view those needs should be defined, from the political, from that of cost-containment, of cost-effectiviness, or that of society.
Wagner: suggested that all the standpoints mentioned by the questioner are parts of the same group: the society.
Vrijland, chairman: proposed, to return to this in the final discussion, since the whole symposium is concerned with this problem.

References

1. Cooperation of Health Care and Education at the Regional Level: Problems, Responsibilities and Cost-allocation. National Seminar in The Netherlands, The Hague, 1978.
2. Jantsch, E (Ed.): Perspectives of Planning: Proceedings of the OECD Working Symposium on Long-Range Forecasting and Planning (Bellagio, Italy, 27th October-2nd November 1968), OECD, Paris, 1969.
3. New Directions in Education for Changing Health Care Systems OECD-CERI Report (Chairman: prof. Bror Rexed), Paris, 1975.
4. Kagenaar, P.F.: Onderwijsplanning als instrument van onderwijsbeleid. In: Pedagogische Studiën, 52 , 1975, pp. 207-217, 239-257.
5. Report of the Committee of Inquiry into the Regulation of the Medical Profession (Chairman: dr A.W. Merrison, F.R.S.), HMSO, London, 1975.
6. Report of the Interdepartmental Committee on Medical Schools (Chairman: Sir William Goodenough), London, 1968.
7. Report of the Royal Commission on Medical Education (Chairman: The Rt. Hon. The Lord Todd, D.SC., F.R.S.), London, 1968.
8. Summary Report of The Graduate Medical Education National Advisory Committee ('GMENAC') (Chairman: prof. Alvin R. Tarlov, M.D.), Volume I, september1980 DHSS-Publication No. (HRA) 81-651, Washington, 1981.
9. Financieel Overzicht van de Gezondheidszorg, waarin opgenomen een raming van de kosten tot 1986. Tweede Kamer, zitting 1981-1982, 17.100 Hfdst. XVII, Nr. 14, Den Haag, Staatsuitgeverij, 1982.
10. Report of the International Conference on Primary Health Care, Alma-Ata, USSR, 6-12 September 1978, WHO-Publication, Geneva, 1978.
11. Intramurale Gezondheidszorg in Nederland, 1972-1978, Centraal Bureau voor de Statistiek (CBS), Den Haag, Staatsuitgeverij, 1980.
12. Stephen, W.J.: Round Table: Primary Medical Care and the Future of the Medical Profession, in: World Health Forum, 2 (3), 1978, pp. 315-331.
13. McNutt, D.R.: GMENAC: Its Manpower Forecasting Frame work, in: American Journal Public Health, *71*, 1981, pp. 1116-1124.
14. Bloom, B.S. and Peterson, O.L.: Physician Manpower Expansionism: a policy review, in: Annals of Internal Medicine, *90*, 1979, pp. 249-256.
15. Querido, A.: The Health Sciences Network, Paper, presented at the 10th Anniversary of the Medical Faculty in McMaster University, Unpublished, 1980.
16. Myers, L.P. and Schroeder, S.A.: Physician Use of Services for the Hospitalized Patient: a Review, with Implications for Cost Containment, in: Milbank Memorial Fund Quarterly/-Health and Society, *59*, 1981, pp. 481-502.
17. Ginzberg, E., Braun, E., Hiestand, D. and Ostow, M: The Expending Physician Supply and Health Policy: The Clouded Outlook, in: Milbank Memorial Quarterly/Health and Society, *59*, 1981, pp. 508-539.

18. Van den Bussche, R. and Reerink, E.: Health Services Requirements in the Education of Health Personnel: the Relationship between Health Needs, Health Services and the Training of Health Manpower: report on a study. WHO, Regional Office for Europe, no formal publication, Copenhagen, 1979.

SESSION II:

REALITIES IN MANPOWER PLANNING IN EUROPE

Medical Manpower Planning in the Federal Republic of Germany

*Mrs M. Schleicher, M.A. Law**

For me the term 'Health Manpower Planning' is above all connected with two main problem areas. One concerns the question 'What kind of manpower is needed in the public health sector?' The other may be summarized as follows: 'How many health personnel do we need? Especially, how high a figure of the staff of the individual health professions is required in order to ensure an adequate health care system covering the whole population?'
All those who deal with these questions know that their examination leads into a vast field which is difficult to explore, they are aware of the manifoldness of the problems occuring in this context which are often difficult to comprehend, and they realize how variable the answers have to be in view of the fact that they have to respond to different situations and that they are determined by differing objectives.

With the required brevity, I shall try to make some comments from the point of view of a country in which the endeavours towards best qualified health professions have been traditional for a long time.

The ranking of a guaranteed level and excellent qualifications of the health professions with us becomes evident through the fact that the Basic Law of the Federal Republic of Germany, in continuance of previous regulations, has assigned to the Federal Government a concurrent legislative authority for conferring the licenses to practise medical and other health professions. It hereby becomes possible to create, for the protection and welfare of the citizen throughout the entire Federal territory, uniform job descriptions and uniform patterns of training which secure a minimum level of qualification. With the license to practise a profession given pursuant to the pertaining laws, the State warrants a guarantee for qualified an properly trained health personnel.

Apart from the licenses of the academic health professions, i.e. physicians, dentists, pharmacists and veterinarians, the Federal Government has also regulated the licenses to practise a profession for midwives (Hebammen), the staff of the nursing professions (Krankenschwestern und

* Unfortunately mrs Schleicher was not able to present her paper at the symposium.

Krankenpfleger, Kinderkrankenschwestern, Krankenpflegehelfer), medical technicians (medizinisch-technische Laboratoriumsassistenten, medizinisch-technische Radiologieassistenten, veterinärmedizinisch-technische Assistenten), physiotherapists (Masseure und medizinische Bademeister, Krankengymnasten), dietitians (Diätassistenten), pharmacy technicians (pharmazeutisch-technische Assistenten), ergotherapists (Beschäftigungs- und Arbeitstherapeuten) and logopedists (Logopäden). In addition to the demands for the moral and physical qualification being the prerequisite for the practice of these professions, these regulations cover the minimum requirements for the respective vocational training. The latter is one of the focal points of these regulations with all professions. Besides the rules governing the sphere of activity and its delimitation, the regulations for the vocational training are decisive for the relevant job description as well as its classification and significance within the comprehensive concept of the health professions.

As it is here where we find the starting point for creating the training patterns adjusted to needs and for formulating the job descriptions, it goes without saying that these regulations are elaborated not only with special care and with the extensive cooperation of the practising professional circles but that they are also subject to a continuous process of observation and adaptation with regard to the changing demands in practice, especially the altered requirements in the health care of the population.

With reference to the subject of the symposium, I consider it important to point out in this connection that, according to our experiences, the majority of the health professions have evolved from practice. These professions developed as a result of a certain demand for care services among the population whereby the general evolution of living conditions as well as advancing findings and opportunities in medicine and the related sciences were of decisive influence. In this country, there was hardly ever any so-called 'planning' of health professions as defined by a draft for the new creation of certain professions, and I wonder if it would make sense to endeavour any such planning within a field which has naturally grown, which is continuing to take shape and which is very dependent on the evolution of general living conditions and the economic situation. Such planning would too easily entail the danger of missing the necessities of practice. This does, however, not mean the abandonment of prospective studies and long-range planning with the health professions. Elements of planning are not only justified but even necessary where it is our job to adapt the individual vocational training patterns of these health professions to present and future needs of care services among the population, to design them as best we can for these purposes and to integrate the very profession appropriately into the context of the rest of the health professions.

An example of the recent past is to illustrate what I have explained on the formation of health professions and on the necessity of checking and steering evolutions in time. As was the case in other countries, the professional groups of the non-medical psychotherapists has emerged here as well. It has developed from practice due to the persisting health care needs, which can be met by means of applying psychotherapeutical methods through staff who are specially qualified. What is to be done now is to integrate this profession, after assessing the future health care needs and the opportunities of meeting them, into the comprehensive spectrum of the health professions and to find a way of training for it which permits to bring it optimally into action within the field of public health. I do not intend to go into detail about the number of difficulties and problems involved and neither do I want to deal with the kind of these difficulties and problems. I think everybody is familiar with them. I am pointing them out to explain that a sensible settlement of this area necessitates a far-sighted way of acting, an assessment of future evolutions as well as their consideration in the programmes. We have always looked upon the full cooperation of everyone concerned as an expedient method of securing a training which is adjusted to the needs and which provides for a reasonable integration into the system of health professions. It is unrenouncable that with such processes – let me call them 'planning processes' in this connection – professional practitioners and representatives of the different government bodies are just as much given a hearing as the professionals and the persons concerned in the educational sector, the experts from research and the specialists from the fields of social security plus the staff dealing with the expenses.

Let me give you another example to explain the practice in our country: with the medical training I want to touch upon a topic which is currently again the object of intensified discussions and careful considerations.

After the criticism of medical training had increased here and the necessity of steps for its improvement had become evident, the responsible Federal Ministry for Youth, Family Affairs and Health had in 1975 coopted a 'ad hoc-Commission on questions of medical training and the future development in the field of the medical profession'. This Commission was made up of both representatives of the responsible Federal ministries and ministries of the Laender, and of representatives of the universities and the medical faculties, the scientific associations, the physicians, the legal health insurance companies, the students and the trade unions. It has comprehensively dealt with the problems of medical training and compiled recommendations which are the basis of the ministry's work for amending the Code regulating the practice of medicine (Approbationsordnung).

It has to be mentioned in passing that this Commission has also examined other fields, made important recommendations for the 'Movement of the number of medical students' and proposals on other topical questions of importance for the advancement in the field of the medical professions such as the 'Role of the physician in general medicine', the 'Role of the physician in health education and information', the 'Working hours of hospital physicians' and on the subject 'Fields of activity of the medical practice with problems of servicing'.

It is common practice with *all* codes regulating the practice of medicine and with *all* regulations on the vocational training and examination that they are prepared on a very broad basis which makes it possible to consider also future servicing needs and the corresponding evolution on the demand side. In this connection it has to be noted that, through the framework set-up by EEC legislation for the vocational training patterns of several health professions, pertaining experiences flow in from within the European Community. After a new regulation on the vocational training and examination of midwives has thus been passed recently, a reform of the vocational training patterns for the nursing professions is now being prepared analogously.

Before I go on to the question as to the quantitative demand for the staff of the individual health profession I want to emphasize that all of us keep the evolution in the field of the health professions under continuous review and are endeavoured to catch up with new progressions in good time.

There are various ways for realizing this. One of it is to try and explore future evolutions and servicing needs by selective research measures. If new job descriptions or a demand for certain services become evident, new courses of training may be tested within the scope of pilot experiments. Currently, such pilot experiments are in progress, e.g. for 'managerial economists in public health' (Betriebswirte im Gesundheitswesen) and for 'engineers in public health' (Ingenieure im Gesundheitswesen). With these professions I am also relating to a development which is typical of the modern field of public health. Changes and advancements in the economic and the technical sector call for experts who have undergone special appropriate education.

It also has to be noticed that there is an ever increasing demand of cooperation with the social professions, as a healthy social environment is the prerequisite for effective preventive, curative and follow-up care. Therefore, we should be and are endeavoured to not only train special professions for public health but also strengthen the willingness and the ability among our health professions to collaborate with other professions as well.

I have extensively dealt with the question concerning the formation of job descriptions and educational training patterns for the health professions, and I have done so on purpose because this is the field where we can best see the opportunities of prospective planning and steering.

The question treating the quantitative demand for the manpower of the individual professions is certainly an important one as well. Where nobody or only few are prepared to choose a profession which is unrenouncable for the community health care, then it is of no use to offer excellent training for this profession. At present, however, we do not face this problem since with all professions in the health sector the demand for places of training courses exceeds by far the number that is available. The number of health professionals has risen in the last few years, for all health professions the figure of the staff actually active in their professions being, however, lower than that of the mere graduates.

Especially among physicians there has been a marked increase of numbers in recent years. Whereas in 1970 the doctor/population ratio was 1 to 612, it already was at 1 to 442 in the year 1980. The evolution featured here is still going to continue over the years to come as with the persistently high number of medical students, some 10,000 to 11,000 graduates are to be expected annually.

There is hardly any point in us asking the question whether so many doctors are really needed. Our Basic Law comprises the principle of the free choice of profession which, according to the practice of constitutional jurisdiction, forbids on principle any system of admission to occupational careers which is adjusted to demand. Any curtailments of the basic right to the free choice of profession may at most become possible in case cardinally important common asset needs to be protected against grave dangers. So as a matter of principle every applicant is to be admitted to the occupational career of own choice as long as suitable training facilities are available or can be created within the scope of economic resources.

Therefore, any planning of the demand for educational training is hardly possible in our country.

Besides, I have the opinion that it is rather difficult to determine the quantitative demand for the stock of the health professions *correctly*. This has been confirmed by various attempts at drawing up analyses of demand with individual nursing professions which were conducted within the scope of research commissions. I do not mean to go into the problems in detail, yet I want to raise the question: what are the *safe* findings on which one might base such estimates at all? For individual fields it may well be possible to establish certain trends. But can such estimates be so comprehensive as to find safe foundations for an analysis of demand with all the decisive factors? Can one assess at the same time what the future health care needs will be like, how diseases and health are going to develop, which course the general conditions of life will take, what health behaviour the individual will assume, which general hopes and expectations will prevail, and which progresses in medicine and the related sciences, and in political economy we have in prospect?

Surely you may find simpler parameters for establishing number of demands. I suppose those countries which have found ways of bringing the admissions to medical training into line with the numbers showing the demand for physicians have not even calculated wrongly in the end.

At any rate it seems important to discuss the chances and limitations of foresight and planning in the field of the health professions also at international level. By mutually exchanging our experiences we can learn a good deal from one another in this domain. And it was at this Symposium where we got the oppurtunity of doing so.

Medical Manpower Planning in The Netherlands

J.M. Greep, M.D.

'Did we come here to laugh or cry?
Are we dying or being born?'
Terra Nostra by Carlos Fuentes

Introduction

'Who needs manpower planning? Is there anything wrong with the figures and facts of health care. Who told you so? There is no problem. The doctors have enough patients, enough work. The demands of the patients are unlimited'. Every problem can be translated into a health problem: 'Doctor please, help, my husband drinks'. Every year thousands of students want to start a medical study. So what are we talking about.

Sure, there are enough patients and there are enough students. The problem is that within the current workload the health manpower resources in The Netherlands are too excessive. The current medical market is exaggerated. Today a small percentage of the health care workers, including general practitioners and specialists are out of work and in view of the planned closure of 15% of all hospital beds, - a recent cost-control measure - more problems will arise. A total of 900 doctors are out of work and registered as such and many more will follow. That is really new. There seems no money available to create new jobs. In medicine new jobs mean new investments in equipment and more health care costs. We are spending already 32 billion guilders. About f 2.300,- for each inhabitant of The Netherlands, sick or healty, yearly.

The principles of continuous progress and continuous growth of the health care industry have been seriously shaken recently. The international financial economic situation is in poor shape. A continuing decline is everywhere visible; the amount of bankruptcies ever increasing. We cannot afford anymore to let things happen. We have to plan in order to avoid a health care bankruptcy. This is not a special Dutch problem. You undoubtedly will hear the same statements from other speakers.

Already in 1977 Newsweek published an article entitled: 'A radical cure for high medical costs'. When one decides to let the costs come to a hold and to fix a budget for the total amount to be spent on health care, it becomes necessary to make decisions on priorities and judge how the money has to be spent. Questions on quality, quantity and accessability of health care have to be answered. If one wants to shift high costs from intramural hospital care to lower costs for extramural general practitioners care – specialist care to general practice and paramedical care, long-term care towards short-term care – it is time to study these complex problems carefully and to make decisions. Plans have to be started according to this. Political decisions have to be made and calculations in terms of manpower will follow. The political ideology is crucial; in a socialistic approach the planning has probably to be more extensive then in a free enterprise system. A socialistic system is undoubtedly more bureaucratic. The expected amount of income of the health care workers plays an important role in all the calculations.

It is a difficult task to develop health manpower planning in a country. Till now in The Netherlands the necessary basic information about health care personnel is not in details available. The exact number of functioning specialists can only be estimated. To develop health manpower planning, many factors have to be considered, such as workload, the market, structure and function of the health care system, the intensity of population coverage, the distribution of personnel, the integration of services, etc.

The Dutch situation

The total cost of health care in The Netherlands has steadily risen from 5% of the Gross National Product (GNP) in 1965, via 8,15% GNP in 1975, till about 10% in 1982. Over 230,000 workers, this is about 6,5% of our total working population, are functioning in our health care system. The cost of wages consists of over 70% of the total health care cost.

Till now there is no health manpower planning in The Netherlands. Don't think that things are easily happening in The Netherlands because it is a small country. Due to a high degree of individuality and freedom we have the habit of dividing ourselves in small groups and sub-groups. Over 100 religions are active. Over 6,000 political parties are registered when town and city councils are elected. In nation-wide elections, 23 political parties are active, of which about 10 reach parliament. 10 Politically and religious connected broadcasting corporations are functioning. This tendency towards independence is possibly the result of our fight with the sea, to keep our homeground safe.

The Health Care System

The health care system looks like a painting of Breugel: many activities all over the place, no priorities, no planning, no control, it works, but we do not know how to handle it.

The system was founded during the German occupation in 1941. Almost 70% of the population is in a 'Krankenkasse' system covered by compulsory health care. The premiums are paid by employer and employee. The non-compulsory insured part of the population is either voluntarily insured within the compulsory program or has a private type of medical insurance. There is a clear division between general practitioners and general hospital specialists. The system is hospital directed and even general practitioners need the stimulus of hospital care by a referral system.

In health care private enterprise prevails but in view of the ever increasing costs government is slowly intervening and new laws are in the making to restructure the health care system and to abandon the 'laissez faire' period. Government is of the opinion that it should get more grip on the system since health is very important to its citizens and the very high life expectancy in our country is now stalling. The first blue print to reform our health care system was made in 1974 by the Secretary of Health mr Hendriks.

Only recently a follow-up to this intention was given with a law called: 'Wet Voorzieningen Gezondheidszorg', a law on health distribution created to get the health care system under control and to start planning on a regional, provincional basis. Until recently the doctors and the hospitals had an enormous freedom but this will end and guidance will be given by the political system of the provinces.

Medical schools

It is our firm belief that we should be concerned with the future and the health care system and medical schools should not be allowed to passively wait for things to happen; we have to be actively involved. This is why we were most pleased when the junior hospital doctors asked us to cooperate with them in the organization of this manpower symposium. Medical schools cannot stay away from taking responsibility. In Maastricht responsibility for an early engagement with the health care system is stressed. So it is natural for the board of the medical school to look outside the ivory tower of medicine.

Some Dutch figures and facts

At the moment 5,350 general practitioners are in function. Many more general practitioners are trained (about 500 yearly) in a one year training program. 2,000 Inhabitants is seen by many as an achievable General Practitioner inhabitant relation figure while in Great Britain already 1,700 is seen as the most ideal figure for the GP's list. The government hopes to strenghten the first line (GP) care. They are stimulating general practitioners to look after more patients outside the hospital in the community.

The specialist field presents a simular problem. In 1982 about 9,000 specialists are in function. Over 600 young specialists are yearly finishing the 29 specialty training programs creating a net increase of about 350-400 specialists on a yearly basis.

With national unemployment now running around 10% the figure of the 0,3% unemployment for general practitioners and specialists sounds heavenly. Even so it means that an appreciatable number of expensively trained highly skilled people are twiddeling their thumbs and rapidly losing their skills. The latest information given shows that about 900 qualified general practitioners and specialists are registered as unemployed by March 1, 1982. We are undoubtedly overtraining and manpower planning is mandatory.

Influences on manpower planning

Population

The population of The Netherlands will grow slowly till about 15 million in the year 2000, passing the 14,5 million mark in 1990. The aging of our population is an important problem. 12-13% Of the population will be over 65 in the next decade. 15% In the year 2000. A person over 65 will be 3 times more often admitted to a hospital than somebody under 65 and many - specialized - nursing homes are necessary for our aging population.

Referrals

In a referral system the amount of referrals is crucial. Referrals are steadily rising (figure 1) although recently a slower increase is seen. At the moment there are about 6.2 million referrals yearly. The increase in 1979 was only 1%.

Referrals 1980

	Number	Referrals
Sickfunds	10 mill.	5 mill.
Private	4 mill.	1.2 mill.
Total	14 mill.	6.2 mill.

Increase 1979 - 1980 1%

Figure 1

Diagnostic Procedures

There is still a growing demand for health care and especially diagnostic procedures are ever increasing. In the period 1975 till 1980 all diagnostic procedures increased by 40%, especially in X-ray diagnosis a 55% increase was seen. By creating diagnostic centres the general practitioners will also have access to the diagnostic possibilities of hospitals. If this will decrease the amount of specialistic help, is an important question but doubtful. A recent example of the profound effect of new technology is the case of the CAT scanner. The scanner's advantages are indisputable but its usefulness has not been carefully evaluated?

Workload

The workload and time per patient will increase. Governmental forces will try to close hospital beds. From 4,7/4,8 beds per thousand population in 1982, to 3,7 beds per thousand population in the next decade. It is difficult to calculate the effect on health manpower. Less specialist positions might be available and about 15,000 nurses have to be retrained. New hospital outpatient facilities are necessary and more general practitioners have to function in the community.

Financial aspects

Many problems, especially financial ones, have to be solved. In The Netherlands most general practitioners and specialists function as free enterprise workers with their own small business. At the end of their productive period they sell their practice for the net of one year production. A kind of build in pension plan; we call it a goodwill system.

If the government wants to control the health care system, the goodwill has to be paid in the form of pensions to the departing doctors or cash to the younger doctors.

Other factors

Many other factors will influence the workload in the future. Increasing democracy will ask more time, more interspecialistic consultation time will be necessary, resultating in more administration and more quality control. In view of this, more time for continuous education, will be necessary. Arbitrarily we have to calculate a 10% increase of this type of workload.

In total all activities due to the population increase, the aging of the population of the everlasting referrals, the increase of the workload, with a decrease of the working time; e.g. 50 hours, a total increase of doctors, up to 25%, might be necessary in the near future.

The essential change required in the next years is the creation of a climate of an organization in which medical education and manpower planning will go hand in hand. The promotion of flexibility in the deployment of manpower is essential and an important factor in helping the country to get value for the health profession money. But first the medical profession and the politicians have to select the best system of health care provision. If the current free enterprise system will change in the direction of a more socialized system with all health care workers employed in a 40 hours working week different calculations are necessary for our health educational planning. The future system of choice has to be brought into consideration.

Manpower of the future

In the following calculations we like to assess the need for general practitioners and specialists considering the current situation and the 50 and 40 hours week options.

For short-term planning the entry in the first year medical school is necessary. To assess these figures a national acceptability is necessary and centralization of the planning mandatory. For a long-term action, c.q. the magic year, 2000 a different approach is required.

Female doctors

More and more female students are seen in the medical faculties. From 25% in 1960 till about 40% in 1981. The amount of female doctors is slowly increasing. About 7% will follow a GP training in 1980 with an expected increase till 12% in 2000. In specialistic programmes, the amount will slowly increase to an estimated 25%. In social health care over 60% of all female doctors will be employed. In total about 20% of functioning doctors will be female.

Manpower planning for general practitioners

Assuming that the current referral system is maintained and assuming that no major financial changes will take place in the direct future, a proportional large amount of single-handed practitioners will continue to function in this system.

Important for the calculations of training positions and the related medical school figures are the ratio GP-inhabitants of a community. The 2,500-2,700 inhabitants to one general practitioner will be used for the short-term calculations. The figure of 2000 inhabitants on one GP list in the year 2000 will be used as the ideal long-term proposition. In figure 2 these figures are presented.

G.P.			
1977	**4926**	**1 : 3000**	**473**
1979	**5692**		**550**
1981	**6700**	**1 : 2000**	**550**
1983	**7700**		

Figure 2

So the growth of general practitioners to one general practitioner for 2,000 inhabitants in the year 2000 needs a continuous inflow of 350 till 400 general practitioners. Taking in consideration that about 80% of all trained general practitioners will finally reach their goal and start a practice, about 400 training positions are necessary in 1983 and about 500 in 1990. The current training, of 550 general practitioners, will create more unemployment.The current unemployed doctors can be used to compensate for the next years; so absolutely no more than 350 training positions (45 for each faculty?) are necessary in the first five till seven years and no more than 350 basic doctors, are necessary to finish the medical school for the GP specialty. Later a maximum of about *425* basic doctors are necessary to be trained in a two-three year GP training programme.

	1981	1985	1990	1995	2000
total GP	5,400	6,300	6,700	6,750	7,800
yearly outflow (3%-4%)	220	220	250	270	270
yearly inflow needed	220	220	250	270	270
yearly needed for expansion	125	125	125	125	125
total inflow	345	345	375	400	400

Figure 3

Manpower planning for specialists

In calculating the necessary total amount of specialists, the calculation of the workload for a working week is mandatory. The general accepted 50-55 hours workweek seems realistic. A 40 hours week is also included in the calculations to please the 'fairy tale tellers' of socialist origin.

In the specialty training programme are 13% female specialists with a productive period of 72% creating a net specialist training production of 96%.

The amount specialists needed in 1983 till the year 2000 can be calculated with the assumption of:

1. a freeze of the current system inflow = outflow
2. a 50-hours week
3. a 40-hours week
4. the current system with an inflow of 600 young doctors yearly with an average training of 4,8 year.

For 1. 220, 2. 350 and 3. 570 basic doctors are necessary for specialist training. In view of the current developments and the overtraining in many specialties, there are in the period 1983 till 1994 a maximum of *350* basic doctors needed for a speciality training. If health care will be nationalized according to the Swedish or British system, about *600* basic doctors are mandatory for training. This will result in over 15,000 specialist in the year 2000! (figure 4).

YEARLY	1981	1990	2000
1. 220 - 250	8,600	8,600	8,600
2. 350	8,600	9,770	11,000
3. 570 - 600	8,600	11,500	14,800
4. 625 (currently)	8,600	12,200	15,600

Figure 4

Manpower planning for the social health care system.

The social health care system needs an additional amount of basic doctors. In 1982 about 30% of all our workers in *industry* have some health care covering during labour hours. In the year 2000 a total of 2,000 labour health doctors are necessary to cover the industrial needs.

Baby-, school-, and youth- health care need many part- time jobs. Especially female doctors are attracted to those positions. In the total field of social health care many doctors in part-time functions can be used.

Incalculating all aspects to social health care, another *130* basic doctors are necessary for these and other types of training programmes.

Other fields

For the training of students and residents many doctors are needed by the medical faculties. For the specialistic and GP fields about 30-40 basic doctors have to be calculated for this type of activity while abount 30-50 are necessary on a yearly basis for research industry, military activities, etc. In calculation all aspects of health care, health economic, military services, etc. another *150* basic doctors are necessary.

All this information should help the department of education to calculate the right amount of medical students necessary for our country.

In The Netherlands free access to the universities has always been a constitutional right. In view of the training limitation of the current medical faculties, *1970* medical students are now allowed (figure 5).

They are admitted by a weighed lottery. The real number of students has never been calculated in relation to the real needs of our society. The introduced manpower related system allows us to calculate the necessary number of students that is allowed to enter our eight medical faculties.

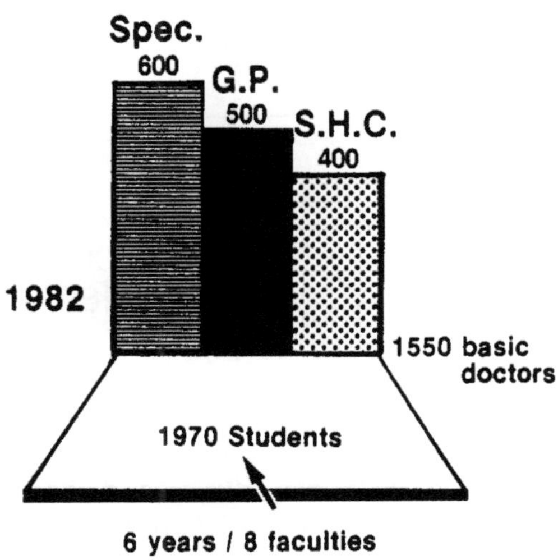

Figure 5

total basic doctors necessary		resulting in		
	1983	1980	1990	2000
general practitioners	350	5,400	6,700	7,800
specialists	350	8,600	9,770	11,000
social health	130	1,000	2,000	3,000
others	240	9,600	10,500	11,300
total	1,070	24,600	28,970	33,100

Figure 6

In view of our current calculations for 1983 (figure 6) only a *1,070* basic doctors are necessary. In view of the fact that about 75%-80% of the medical students will reach this goal about *1,200* medical students should be allowed to enter Dutch medical schools (figure 7).

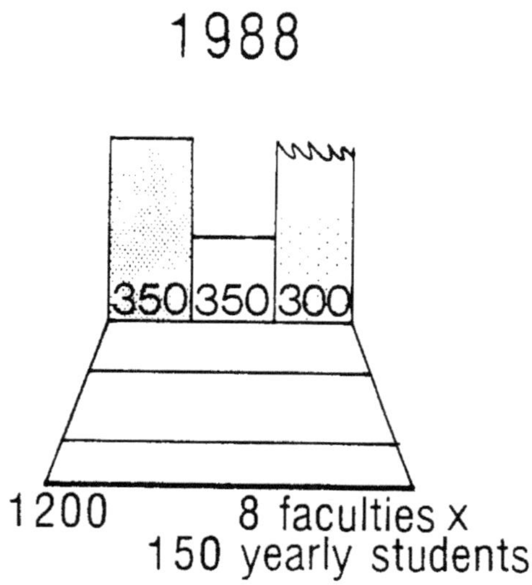

Figure 7

Many students will try to find training posts inside The Netherlands or mainly in a Common Market Country, during and after their study many will return to the Dutch market, but in view of the fact that no real figures are available, re-adjustments have to be made in the future using the real figures.

Besides the Dutch foreign production about 800 foreign doctors are working in The Netherlands, 50% are from the European Community.

There is a great desirability of integrating the health manpower planning with the total health education system. The planning of the number of physicians and the planning of nurses and paramedical manpower has to be integrated. Other social health systems with training, in prevention, management, health care economics, epidemiology, etc., have to be brought in tune with doctor's manpower studies.

Protocols

We are on the brink of starting a health manpower planning programme in The Netherlands. For cost control it is fundamental to connect this planning with epidemiological studies and with protocols for the function of general practitioners and specialists. These protocols have to be used to increase the efficiency of medical intervention and to create a system of quality control.

The future

Some problems are created by the desirability for a 40 hours week. Can The Netherlands economy afford over 7,000 GP and over 15,000 specialists? In view of this calculation the workload of the female doctor in the system can also create a problem. Despite these and other problems we know that there is an urgent need for short term planning and action in view of the rising unemployment rate of physicians. At the moment we are mopping our wet floors while the faucets are running. We have to stop these faucets. The first year medical school is the year where manpower planning should start today.

Medical Manpower Planning in France

E. Duchene, M.D.

To start with, I would like to point out that I shall only be talking about planning for doctors and not for auxiliary or paramedical staff.

I would like to deal with medical planning from two different angles.

Access to medical studies and access to establishment. As regards access to establishment we must say immediately that establishment is in theory totally free in France. This is correct as far as independent practice is concerned, but we should bear in mind on the one hand the problems of vacant positions in public establishments and on the other hand, the difficulty of finding a satisfactory post in private clinics for the exercise of certain specialities. Those are material and practical contingencies which do not result from a legal requirement.

The situation is different for access to medical studies; during previous governments it was in fact thought necessary to provide for a selection procedure in France within the framework of medical studies in order to cope with medical population problems and in order to ensure that training would be as much as possible in accordance with the necessary quality requirements and criteria, particularly in the European field. In fact, from 1963 to 1973 the number of students in their first year of medicine tripled, rising from 10,000 to 34,500. Also the number of those who obtained a medical qualification rose from 3,504 in 1970 to 9,186 in 1977.

The total number of practising doctors in July 1979 was 97,314 (of those 17,139 were women).

Therefore, in 1979 the density was 200 doctors per 100,000 inhabitants (against 129 in 1970 and 156 in 1975). On January 1st 1980 there were 116,104 doctors registered with the Panel of the Order (of those 24,722 were women).

On December 31st 1980, there were 124,370 doctors registered at the Panel of the Order (of those 27,178 were women).

On April 1st 1981, there were 128,275 doctors registered at the Panel of the Order.

We have had to note, therefore, that the number of doctors is increasing.

According to the report, which the minister, M. Barrot, asked professor Etienne to draw up, if the growth of the medical student population is not curbed, the number of doctors would double by the year 2000, and the

NUMBERS OF MEDICAL STUDENTS IN FRANCE

source: the ministry of National Education of France

academic years		63-64	64-65	65-66	66-67	67-68	68-69	69-70	70-71
first part	1st year	9,990	11,750	12,920	14,600	21,060	25,690	25,530	25,360
	2nd year	3,460	6,220	7,540	8,870	10,100	14,730	15,730	12,500
second part	1st year	6,710	3,480	4,920	5,880	7,050	8,200	12,240	11,500
	2nd year	4,130	5,450	3,400	4,520	5,350	6,000	8,220	11,500
	3rd year	3,490	3,920	5,110	3,860	4,740	6,240	6,750	8,000
	4th year	2,870	3,370	3,590	4,610	3,550	4,880	4,880	6,500
	total ---	17,200	16,220	17,020	18,870	20,690	25,320	32,090	37,500
third part (certificated)		2,930	2,800	3,370	3,480	4,600	3,420	4,190	4,500
general total ---------		33,590	36,990	40,860	45,820	56,440	69,160	77,540	82,500

Figure 1 Until selection was started: from 1963 to 1971

academic years		71-72	72-73	73-74	74-75	75-76	76-77	77-78	78-79	79-80
first part	1st year	29,000	30,700	34,500						
	2nd year	13,500	10,500	10,000	9,500					
second part	1st year	11,000	11,000	9,500	9,500	9,500				
	2nd year	11,500	11,000	11,000	9,500	9,200	9,200			
	3rd year	11,500	11,500	11,000	11,000	9,500	9,000	9,000		
	4th year	8,000	11,500	11,500	11,000	11,000	9,500	9,000	9,000	
	total ---	42,000	45,000	43,000	41,000	39,200				
third part (certificated)		6,500	8,000	11,500	11,500	11,000	11,000	9,500	9,000	9,000
general total ---------		91,000	94,200	99,000						

Figure 2 After selection was started: from 1971 to 1980 (date of diploma for students registered with the PCEM, 1973-1974) - (provisional figures)

medical density would then go from 182 to 300 practitioners per 100,000 inhabitants. At the same time, on the 30th of November 1980 we found that unfortunately there were doctors in need of a job, as 1,704 unemployed doctors were registered at the National Employment Agency.

In this respect we want to show you the following statistics which come from the ministry for National Education (figures 1 and 2).

So a procedure was envisaged, not upon admission to the first year, but at the end of the first year of the first part of the study of medicine.

The selection procedure aimed to achieve better training of students within the framework of European standards. It's object was also to limit medical unemployment, if possible.

It was provided, therefore, that the ministers concerned - at the time these were the ministers for Health and the Universities - would determine the number of students in the first year of the first part of the study of medicine who would be admitted to entry into the second year of the first part.

This decision was to be taken annually based on the following criteria:

- due consideration of the needs of the population;
- the need to comply with certain training standards: in respect of the ratio between the number of students and the number of teachers and between the number of students and the training bodies. This results in the obligation to obtain a better distribution over the various universities in order to avoid untimely flow towards certain training centres.

The whole of this system was organized by an Act of July 12th 1979, which also included transitional measures.

It was, in fact, decided that for the two academic years following this Act of 1979 the variation of overall numbers of students permitted to continue their studies after the first year of the first part should not exceed ten percent of the total number compared to the previous year. For the academic year 1980/1981 the number of first year studies was set at 6,409 (instead of 7,121 for the year 1979/1980) and the target for 1983 was the figure of 5,000 students. At present, however, in view of the change in direction which has ocurred in France, it is no longer certain that the selection system will be maintained. The reforms stipulated for 1983 after ten years of work on medical studies and put into concrete terms by the Act of 6th July 1979 are deferred until 1984.

The new government thinks now that the existing provisions should be changed and that 'true reform means bringing hospital facilities up to their teaching standards and, also to bring about total renewal of the teaching methods of the first two parts of the medical studies' syllabus in order to prepare students and to direct them towards general practice, research, public health or a career as a specialist'.

For the year 1981/1982, the two ministers concerned have decided to maintain numbers at the same level as for 1980/ 1981, that is: 6,409. On the other hand, the reduction provided for by the Act of 1979 and its implementing legislation is not continued.

It is not up to me to pronounce judgement on how well-founded the development is which has been started. I will just state some of the reactions we hear at the present time. The medical profession itself in France would tend to prefer maintaining some selection.

This is why the 'Confédération des Syndicats Médicaux Français' was prompted to state that 'In view of the attraction of medical studies we wish for selection. All statistics show that the level of work of practitioners is diminishing. Professional people cannot be trained indefinitely without being offered places afterwards. Health education or school medicine cannot offer the necessary employment on their own. With numbers as high as 6,500 or 7,000 students a year, medical density will continue to grow until the year 2000. Only a numerus clausus, varying according to the facilities, could make up for regional imbalances'.

Much the same thing is said by the National Association of Medical Students in France and the Federation of French Doctors: 'Demography is the major problem. We have sufficient doctors to allow satisfactory health cover of the country. It is a question of information but also of incentive measures, financial, fiscal or any other type . . .'

The National Order of Doctors, also basing itself solely on the point of view of the quality of doctors and their training, has for a long time, been in favour of applying certain rules in this respect.

Finally, in the recent report by the Investigating Committee on Training and Scientific Development, professor Laurent Schwartz, member of the Institute, appears to pinpoint a lack of balance between the proposed training schemes and existing needs. He thus attributes some merit to the principle of selection upon entry into university, whilst at the same time he also takes account of the necessary equality of chances.

This then is the present situation in France, a situation which is evolving and changing all the time, as you can see. You will, therefore, understand, that I cannot be more precise than I have been.

Medical Manpower Planning in the United Kingdom

Michael E. Abrams, M.D.

In the United Kingdom the government sets the medical school student intake at an appropriate level so as to ensure that the future supply of UK trained doctors will be adequate. It is generally accepted that the number of places in British medical schools should be set in accordance with the best estimate that can be made of the number of doctors the country will wish to employ in future years. The Health Departments undertake this planning work and in doing so have to take account of the possible future needs of all branches of medicine both within the National Health Service (general practice, hospital and community medicine); in the public sector, for instance, universities and research councils; in the private sector, such as industry including the pharmaceutical industry and occupational medicine; solely private practitioners; the armed forces and government, etc. It takes, by the nature of medical training in the UK, some 9 to 16 years from a student entering medical school to his taking up a career post in one of these branches of medicine. Thus, the decisions affecting the number of doctors trained in the UK who will be available for medical work over the next 10 years or so have already been made. To take a view about the number of medical students we should train in the future we have therefore to make projections about the likely demands for doctors at about the end of the century; some 20 years ahead.

Imprecision and uncertainty are inevitable in making such projections. Indeed, purportedly making such calculations precise would be bound to be suspect. We cannot for instance know what proportion of public expenditure or gross national product will be devoted to health care over the next 20 years, or how these resources will be spent, or what changes will take place in the demand for health services and the pattern of health care delivery. Estimates of the numbers of overseas doctors who will continue to come to the United Kingdom are fraught with difficulty. Similarly with the rising number of women now entering medical school we cannot know the extent to which their commitment to medicine will be significantly affected by domestic reponsibilities. In practice therefore we have to work on the basis of the best assumptions we can make knowing that these may have to be changed to reflect unanticipated developments. Implicit in this is that we have regularly to repeat the projections on the basis of the latest information. The UK Health Departments have undertaken such reviews for many years and in 1978 published a Green Paper ('Medical Manpower – the next Twenty Years') whilst in 1980 the DHSS in conjunction with the Treasury and the government's Central Policy Review Staff set up a Steering Group 'to coordinate studies of the supply of and demand for medical manpower in relation to the likely availability of resources up to the end of the century, and to prepare a report'.

Their report was published in 1980; it included a number of different approaches to make the best possible estimates of the demand for and supply of medical manpower up to the year 2000.

Demand

The demand for health services unconstrained by finance appears to be virtually unlimited. Resource availability is therefore probably the most important factor in determining the size of demand in practice and in the past the growth of medical manpower in the NHS has been closely linked with the finance available; which finance comes from the government through general taxation.

The starting point for a financial appraisal must be assumptions about trends in gross domestic product and public expenditure – NHS expenditure currently comprising some 94% of total expenditure on health care. These assumptions are not easy to make; much uncertainty surrounds the future relationship between gross domestic product and total public expenditure with even greater uncertainty attached to the relation between the gross domestic product and any particular expenditure programme. The calculations which follow are thus not predictions of the future, they are illustrative projections of a range of possibilities on which it seems reasonable to base judgment about the effect of demand for medical manpower in the years to come. The Group in 1980 based its resource projections on annual growth rates overall of 1,5% and 2% a year for the Health and Personal Social Services programme so as to estimate the finances which might be available for the various services within the programme.

These overall provisional growth rates for the Health and Personal Social Service programme as a whole have to be further examined so as to estimate growth rates in the hospital and community health services. Further assumptions have to be made here but the conclusion was that growth rates of 1% and 1,4% in the hospital and community health services might for medical manpower planning purposes be taken as the long-term resource assumption arising from 1,5% to 2% growth in the HPSS programme overall. Translating these growth rates for expenditure into provisional projections for medical manpower growth involves further assumptions. The two that were used are

Table 1 Illustrative projection of growth within the HPSS programme - England £ million survey 1979 prices

1980-1981 (I)		1999 to 2000 1½% pa (II)	1999 to 2000 2 % pa (II)
7,647	total overall	10,150	11,140
	personal social services		
1,006	current expenditure at 2% pa	1,460	
	current expenditure at 3% pa		1,760
60	capital expenditure as constant percentage of revenue	85	105
1,350 (III)	family practitioner services (demand led)		
	a) general dental services	280	280
	b) general ophthalmic services	50	50
	c) general medical services		
	list size 2,000) estimated list size 1,800		
	d) pharmaceutical services		
	at 3 % pa at 4½% pa	1,230 or 1,630	1,230 or 1,630
	hospital and community health services		
4,521	current at 1 % pa	5,460	
	current at 1.4% pa	or 5,890	5,890
	current at 2 % pa		or 6,590
370	capital at ca8% of revenue	450	
	capital at ca9% of revenue		550
295	services financed centrally at 0.5% pa	320	320
	total of components	9,805 to 10,635 (IV)	10,715 to 11,815 (V)

(I) net expenditure plans based on Cmnd 7841

(II) average rate of growth in HPSS programme

(III) incorporates adjustment to take account of increased charges announced in Cmnd 7841

(IV) the lower figure assumes that pharmaceutical services grow at 3% per annum and HCH current expenditure grows at 1% per annum. The higher figure assumes that pharmaceutical services grow at 4½% per annum and HCH current expenditure at 1.4% per annum

(V) the lower figure assumes that pharmaceutical services grow at 3% per annum and that HCH current expenditure grows at 1.4% per annum. The higher figure assumes that the pharmaceutical services grow at 4½% per annum and that HCH current expenditure grows at 2% per annum

Table 2 Estimated demand for doctors (I) in the NHS in 2000 based on expected available resources - (Great Britain)

	1978 (actual)		projection assumption	projected demand implied 2000
	27,200	general medical services	average list size 2,000	30,700
			average list size 1,800	34,100
	40,900	hospital and community health service	average annual growth (II) at 1 %	50,900
			average annual growth at 1.5%	56,700
			average annual growth at 2 %	63,200
total demand	68,100	GP list size 2,000	HCH average annual growth (II) at 1 %	81,600
			HCH average annual growth at 1.5%	87,400
			HCH average annual growth at 2 %	93,900
		GP list size 1,800	HCH average annual growth at 1 %	85,000
			HCH average annual growth at 1.5%	90,800
			HCH average annual growth at 2 %	97,300

(I) includes numbers for general medical practitioners and whole-time equivalents for permanent and locum hospital/community health service doctors

(II) average annual growth rates in doctor numbers

a) doctor numbers grow at the same rate of expenditure,
b) within the assumed overall rate of volume growth doctor numbers continue as in the past to grow faster than expenditure.

For general practitioners alternative assumptions of average list sizes of 2,000 and 1,800 were used. The results of these projections are shown in tables 1 and 2.

Case Studies

So as to supplement these demand projections based on resource assumptions the Group examined three areas of the Health Service in England and Wales in order to illustrate some important points about the demand for doctors and the uncertainties and difficulties of forward planning in the field of medical manpower. The areas – obstetric and gynaecology services and services for the elderly and the mentally ill – were chosen because they were affected by contrasting demographic trends. All three studies which do not, and were not intended to, give a comprehensive picture of the NHS, were however of considerable illustrative value. They showed that in these three very different areas patient demand for fully trained doctors has not been met and is likely to increase. This increased demand for doctors results from the continued pressures exerted by both the public and those working in the Health Service to improve the quality of health care as well as from population increases.

Supply

Having estimated the likely future demand for doctors in the NHS the Group then calculated the likely future supply of doctors in order to compare the two sets of projections. Two of the greatest uncertainties in the calculations for the likely future stock arise in connection with the future numbers of overseas doctors coming to the UK and the extent which the increasing number of women doctors will commit themselves to medicine when faced with domestic responsibilities as well.

The Department's Green Paper included projections for the future stock of British and Irish born civilian doctors likely to be active in medicine inside and outside the NHS up to the year 2000. The assumptions used to derive the projections set out in that paper were:

a) there would be 4,080 medical school places in Great Britain from 1983 of which 50% would be occupied by women from 1985;
b) women doctors would be active for 36 years on average (equivalent to 27 years whole-time work) at the beginning of the period and their contribution would increase to 39 years on average (equivalent to 30 years

whole-time work) at the end; net emigration would be at the level of 0,6% of the current stock (equal to 380 per annum from the beginning of the period), and

c) fewer than 25% of doctors over the age of 65 would be active at the beginning of the period and that this proportion would drop to 12% at the end.

These calculations were made in terms of the estimated numbers of active civilian doctors and so as to be able to compare these figures with the estimated levels of demand, the Group expressed them in terms of whole-time equivalents which would be devoted to the National Health Service.

Table 3 Estimated future 'supply' of United Kingdom and Eire born doctors in the NHS in Great Britain

	projection year
	2000
projected stock of GB-born doctors active in medicine (numbers) (I)	83,600
projected stock of Irish-born doctors active in medicine (numbers) (II)	2,150
total (numbers)	85,750
projected stock of active doctors in NHS (whole-time equivalents) (III)	
at 75% of total active stock	64,300
at 80% of total active stock	68,600
at 85% of total active stock	72,900
at 90% of total active stock	77,200

(I) source: table 5 "Medical Manpower - the next 20 years"

(II) source: table 6 "Medical Manpower - the next 20 years"

(III) whole-time equivalent for hospital and community health doctors.
Numbers for general medical practitioners

The factor used was based on DHSS statistics which showed that the ratio of whole-time equivalents of British and Irish born doctors working in the NHS to the total number of active such doctors was about 8 to 10. A range of factors (from ,75 to ,9) was used in the calculations but the range ,8 to ,85 was regarded as the most realistic assumption with the lower end seeming more likely to be realized (table 3).

Projecting the likely migration of overseas qualified doctors is extremely difficult. In the past somewhere in the region of 2,500 to 4,500 such doctors have entered the country each year and about 80% to 85% leave again though not necessarily within the same year. It seems likely for a number of reasons, including the effects of the Medical Act 1978, the attitudes of other countries both to the emigration of their native doctors and the immigration of foreign doctors together with the build-up of postgraduate training facilities elsewhere, particularly in Third World countries that the numbers of overseas doctors coming to the country will fall in the future. It was therefore felt that the most likely assumption was that the stock of overseas doctors in the country would fall over the projection period. Three assumptions were in fact made for the projections – a higher assumption that the *stock* remains constant in the long-term, a medium assumption that it decreases to 70% in the long-term, a low assumption that it decreases to 50% in the long-term. These assumptions gave a very wide range for predicted stock in the year 2000 – from 7,400 to 14,800 with the most likely assumption being 10,400 (table 4). Clearly, when dealing with a total doctor stock in the NHS of some 80,000 these are highly significant figures and it is an area which requires the closest scrutiny in the coming years.

Nearly 1,700 women entered medical schools in Great Britain in 1981 (43% of the total) compared with 523 in 1963 (24%). It is estimated that as many as 50% of new medical students may be women by 1985 – some medical schools have indeed already reached such a proportion. Hence, by the 1990's some half of all new doctors could be women and there would clearly be a marked effect on the proportion of women in the total doctor stock. In comparison, in the ten years up to 1974 the percentage of active doctors under 65 in Great Britain who were women rose only from 19% to some 25%. As the proportion of doctors who are women rises, uncertainty about the future level of their activity rates becomes an increasingly important part of calculations about future stocks of medical manpower. It is clearly not possible to predict how attitudes to combining work and family commitments will change; but if past trends are anything to go by it seems likely that women doctors activity rates will continue to rise as they have for the past 10 to 15 years. For instance, our latest figures show that the proportion of women who are now active in medicine is about 83% compared to 66% in 1965. By contrast the proportion of active male doctors has remained constant at about 88%. A further factor that has to be taken into account is whether the women doctors will in the future be working part-

Table 4 Estimated future supply of overseas-born doctors in the NHS in Great Britain

projected stock of overseas doctors in the NHS (WTEs)	estimated stock 1978 (WTEs)	1980	2000
born and qualified overseas			
medium assumption: stock decreases to 70% in the long-term	13,856	14,800	10,400
high assumption: stock remains constant in the long-term	13,856	14,800	14,800
low assumption: stock decreases to 50% in the long-term	13,856	14,800	7,400
born overseas, qualified in UK or Eire			
medium assumption: stock remains constant at 1978 level	4,700	4,700	4,700
high assumption: stock increases at a level 50% higher than 1978 in the long-term	4,700	4,700	7,000
low assumption: stock decreases to a level 50% of 1978 in the long-term	4,700	4,700	2,400
totals			
medium assumptions	18,556	19,500	15,100
high assumptions	18,556	19,500	21,800
low assumptions	18,556	19,500	9,800

Notes:

The stock of overseas qualified doctors is assumed to rise between 1978 and 1980 because it is assumed that the full effect of the Medical Act will not be felt until 1981. The increase between the two years assumes an annual increase of 3.3% (the estimated average annual growth of these doctors 1975 to 1978) time or whole-time in the Health Service. The trends here are changing but it would appear that there is a tendency for women doctors increasingly to work part-time in the training grades but to increase the contribution which they make while working part-time. It is extremely difficult to quantify these changes but from very tentative calculations it would appear that if women doctors accounted for 50% of all doctors and their activity rates rose to equal those of their male colleagues rather than remaining at their present levels the resultant extra medical input would be equivalent to approximately 2,000 extra doctors. It is clear that the recent rapid increase in the number of women doctors has introduced a new element of uncertainty to long-term medical manpower planning.

Conclusions

These examinations of the demand for and supply of medical manpower make clear that there is a wide unavoidable range of uncertainties in making projections of this kind. On the demand side there are difficulties in attempting to predict the future relationship between the size of gross domestic product and health expenditure and between the latter and expenditure on medical manpower. Although we have used past trends as a basis for our projections we recognize that these may not continue in the future and that the pattern of delivery of health care may change. Turning to the figures themselves at the lower end of the range of projections for the year 2000 we might expect a demand for 81,600 doctors in the NHS in Great Britain. At the upper end the projections give a figure of 97,300. Thus the level of projected demand at the upper end is approximately 20% higher than that of the lower end; our 'best guess' in this range was between 87,400 and 90,800.

On the supply side the greatest uncertainties relate to the future numbers of overseas born doctors, including the long-term effects of the EC-Directives. The assumptions we have had to make in the projections are necessarily crude, but they are crucial, since changes in them would be sufficient to move the supply/demand equations from surplus to shortfall or vice versa. The uncertainties affecting the future stock of British and Irish born doctors are also significant. Different assumptions about the percentage of active medical time devoted to the NHS vary from the low end of the range of assumptions to the high end by some 20%. Whilst a further uncertainty on the supply side is that there will be slower progress towards achieving the medical school target intake of 4,080 places than that envisaged in the projections. This could reduce the supply of UK born doctors by up to 1,800 doctors by the year 2000. Thus amongst the factors affecting these projections, the most critical are the level of demand for doctors in the National Health Service (which depends largely on the financial resources available), the proportion of all medical time devoted by doctors to the National Health Service and the supply of overseas born doctors. Also significant are the uncertainties surrounding the future size of the medical school intake. Although we are most conscious of these uncertainties, we have compared the estimates of demand with the estimates of total supply. This allows a table to be constructed showing the projected shortfall or surplus of doctors in the NHS in the year 2000 based on different assumptions about their activity rates, the growth in the hospital and community health programme and the average general practitioner list size (table 5).

The uncertainties to which these projections are subject have confirmed our view that calculations of this kind must be updated regularly so that the assumptions made can be checked against changes in practice and altered

Table 5 Projected total shortfall or surplus of doctors in the NHS in 2000 AD (Great Britain) (Whole-time equivalent)

	alternative assumptions about the participation rates in the NHS of all active UK and Eire born doctors (i.e. adjustment factor*)			
	75%	80%	85%	90%
a) no growth	+ 11,300	+ 15,600	+ 19,900	+ 24,200
b) GP list size at 2,000				
HCH at 1 % pa	- 2,200	+ 2,100	+ 6,400	+ 10,700
HCH at 1.5% pa	- 8,000	- 3,700	+ 600	+ 4,900
HCH at 2 % pa	- 14,500	- 10,200	- 5,900	- 1,600
c) GP list size of 1,800				
HCH at 1 % pa	- 5,600	- 1,300	+ 3,000	+ 7,300
HCH at 1.5% pa	- 11,400	- 7,100	- 2,800	+ 1,500
HCH at 2 % pa	- 17,900	- 13,600	- 9,300	- 5,000

Notes:

+ = surplus

- = shortfall

* = see text

Overseas doctors:

To simplify this table only the "best guess" medium assumption for overseas-born doctors has been used here. It should be kept in mind that the high and low assumptions would alter the figures quoted here by + 6,700 or - 5,300 respectively where necessary. The Health Departments have kept the medical manpower position under continuing review for many years, and the need for this is illustrated by the fact that since the Green Paper was published in 1978 there has already been a departure from the planned medical school intake. Undoubtedly, there will be further changes over the coming years which should be reflected in projections of this kind. The next such review will be starting later in 1982 by an expert advisory group whose remit will be to provide ministers with advice about the likely demand for medical manpower to enable them to make informed decisions on the appropriate level of medical school intake. The actual terms of reference of this Group are 'within guidelines as to the resources likely to be available to the Health Service to advise the Health Departments upon factors relevant to the government's decision about the appropriate future level of medical school intake in Great Britain including in particular consideration of the most likely range of assumptions about I future demand for doctors both within and outside the NHS; II possible changes in the supply of doctors and including patterns of activity, participation and retirement; III possible changes in migration flows from and to Great Britain'.

References

Medical Manpower, - the next Twenty Years, Her Majesty's Stationery Office, London 1978.

Medical Manpower Steering Group Report, Department of Health and Social Security, London 1980.

Medical Manpower Planning in Sweden

A. Milton, M.D.

As an introduction a brief outline of the institutional framework of the health care and educational systems in Sweden is presented.

Practically all hospitals are publicly owned in Sweden, i.e. owned and operated by one of the 26 county councils. The councils not only provide inpatient, hospital care but are also responsible for approximately 85% of outpatient care - leaving 15% for private practice. The council health services are supervised by central government via its National Board of Health and Welfare but are fairly economically independent due to their right to levy taxes.

In total about 90% of the Swedish medical profession is employed by the counties. The remainder is engaged in private practice or company run health services. Brief and basic facts thus being established about the health system - let's look at the organization of medical training.

Selection of medical students is entrusted to a central board of entrance. The six individual universities do not decide themselves which students will enter their particular medical school. There is also a numerus clausus. Currently 1,026 students start medical studies each year. After 5½ years, 900-950 graduate from medical school ready to start their clinical training of rotating internship lasting 21 months. When this is completed, a full licence to practice as doctors is granted. Practically all fully licenced doctors do, however, countinue to train for a speciality (general practice being one speciality) for another 4½-5 years. Since both systems are decidedly centralized one might wonder about the degree of coordination between the two of them.

To answer that question one first has to recognize that the Swedish economy until recently has been expanding fairly rapidly over the last 30 years. This has been reflected in a very rapid increase in demand, i.e. public demand for medical services. To cope with this rising demand, government multiplied the number of students at the medical faculties several times during the '50's and '60's to the present level of 1,026 students - reached in 1972.

Consequently the medical profession expanded from around 6,000 in 1960 to 18,000 in 1980. Between 1980 and the year 2000 the number will double to an expected 32,000, i.e. more or less one doctor per 250 inhabitants. The expansion of public health care has thus been decisive in determining the dimension of the medical education.

How then have decisions on the strategy of the health care system, i.e. inpatient/hospital versus outpatient care and case oriented versus profylactic health care, influenced allocation of doctors geographically and between specialities/general practice?

Traditionally the process of allocation of doctors has been under strict control by the National Board of Health and Welfare. No positions, whether senior or training, can be created without the approval of the board. In fact all decisions concerning this allocation have been the result of a 'negotiating process' between the Board, the association of county councils and the Swedish Medical Association. The basis for these deliberations have been the long-term health care plans that each county council has adopted. These plans have then been compiled and compared to present day situation with regard to specialist and geographic availability of doctors. With this in mind, plans for the coming 4-5 years have been drawn up, generally with the consent of all parties concerned. Under an expanding economy the problem of medical manpower planning in Sweden has basically been a problem of how to spread scarce resources as evenly as possible. Today there are 900 senior positions vacant. The unfilled vacancies are however unevenly distributed geographically and speciality-wise.

The situation is, however, rapidly changing. Instead of a growth rate of county council health care expenditures at around 4% annually, county councils are now planning for a maximum increase of 1% per year during the next 5-10 years. Any degree of earlier understanding between the medical profession, the employers and the National Board of Health and Welfare in regard to manpower planning has now evaporated. It has not been possible to achieve a long-term planning cooperation between the parties concerned that takes the changing economic outlook into account.

To cope with that, the Swedish Medical Association recently published a manpower prognosis on its own. The Association has done so before and has been heavily criticized when it pleaded against increasing the number of medical students during the '50's, because of a fear of unemployment. In earlier studies the Association tried to estimate the needed number of doctors by seeking an optimal relationship between the number of patients per doctor. That method of course by a wide margin underestimated the demand for doctors - mainly due to the fact that it was impossible to imagine the economic progress and the political, scientific and organizational changes that have taken place during the last 20-30 years.

To avoid falling into the same trap once again, the Medical Association this time used a different and - as we see it - more realistic approach. Basically we started by studing the supply of doctors up to the year 2020 under different assumptions concerning drop out percentages, duration of studies, age of students at study start, etc.

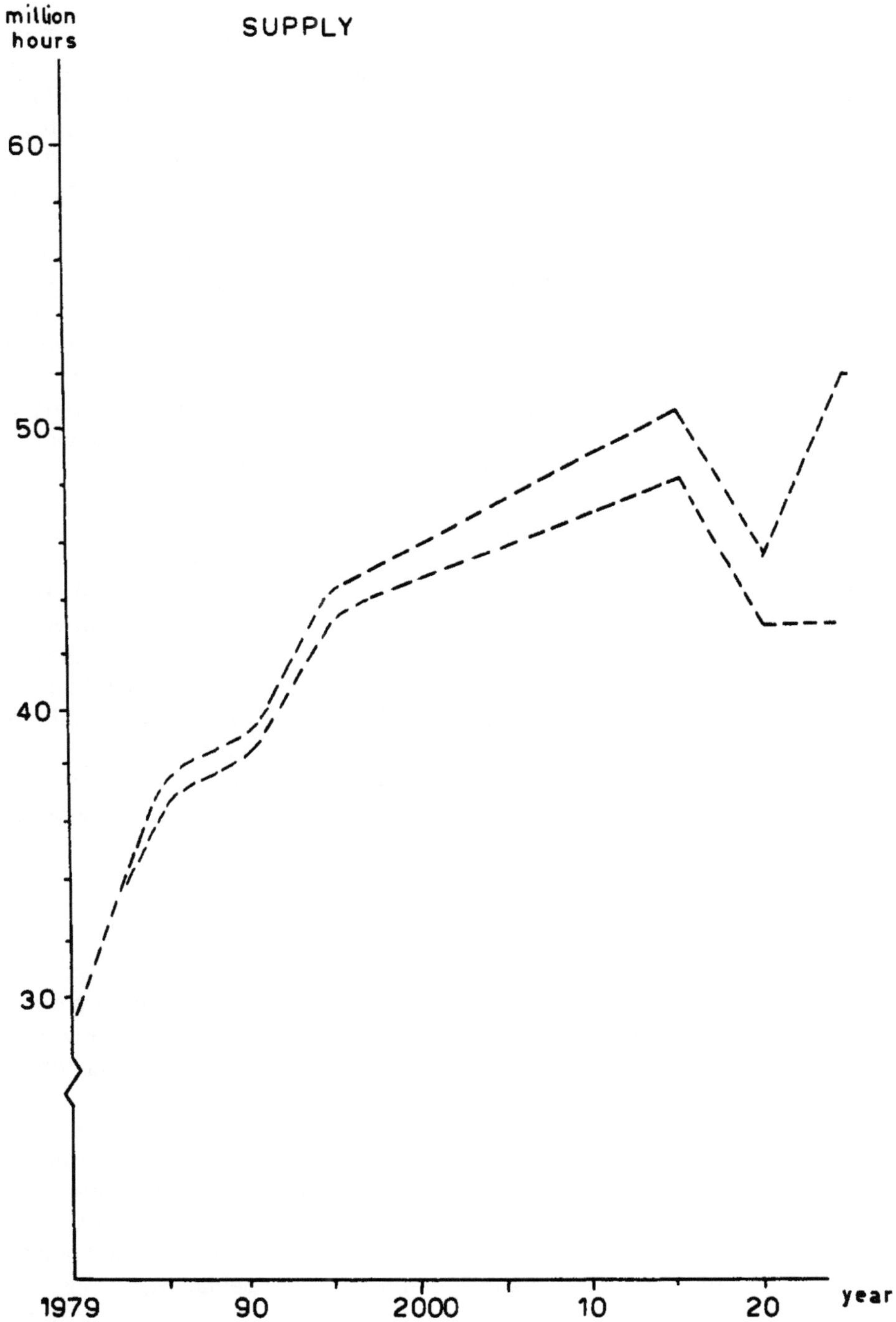

Figure 1

The result can be shown as in figure 1.

As you can see, our assumptions exhibit a maximum and a minimum alternative and for practical reasons the supply is calculated in millions of working hours. The decrease in supply after the year 2015 is a result of the sudden shift of the average age of students starting medical studies from 1977 and onwards. Due to a university entrance reform, the average age at study start increased from 22 to 28 years. Later on the average age of students has decreased to around 25 years.

In order to assess the long-term public demand for doctors, we decided to relate demand to the rate of growth of the Swedish GNP. Knowing the fraction of the GNP today spent on health care and the elasticity of county council growth in relation to growth of the GNP, it is fairly simple with a number of assumptions of course, to calculate public demand for doctors. The crucial point is the nature of the assumptions made - for example the assumption that the number of doctors in relation to other personnel will be fairly constant in spite of a changing role for doctors. The result is shown in figure 2.

Here again we have calculated with a maximum and a minimum alternative and expressed demand in millions of working hours. The maximum level assume a growth rate for demand of 2,4% annually. The lower alternative a rate of growth of 1%. Unfortunately this is the level that the government has asked the county councils not to exceed and a level councils are now reassessing long-term plans to meet. Thus as can be seen in figure 3 supply exceeds demand during the rest of the century for both alternatives and, to the best of our understanding we will see unemployed doctors in Sweden as soon as in the end of the '80's if the economy does not improve to permit county council expenditures on health care to grow with at least 3% annually.

General Discussion

Brearley Sr: suggested that the Dutch and the English situations are quite similar in that there are too few career specialist-posts for too many trainee-specialists. He would like to hear Greeps thoughts on how this imbalance is being tackled in Holland.

Greep: the problem is not entirely analogous. The Dutch private practitioners' income is being reduced through the establishment of norm-incomes. He may be reluctant to share his practice with a new colleague. This reduces his income further while his overheads remain (e.g. 'buying-in' fees). Thus the situation is more complicated than in a nationalized health system and results at this time in 200 unemployed specialists.

A lady-questioner: is there a tendancy for male-doctors to work part-time in England, like female doctors frequently do?

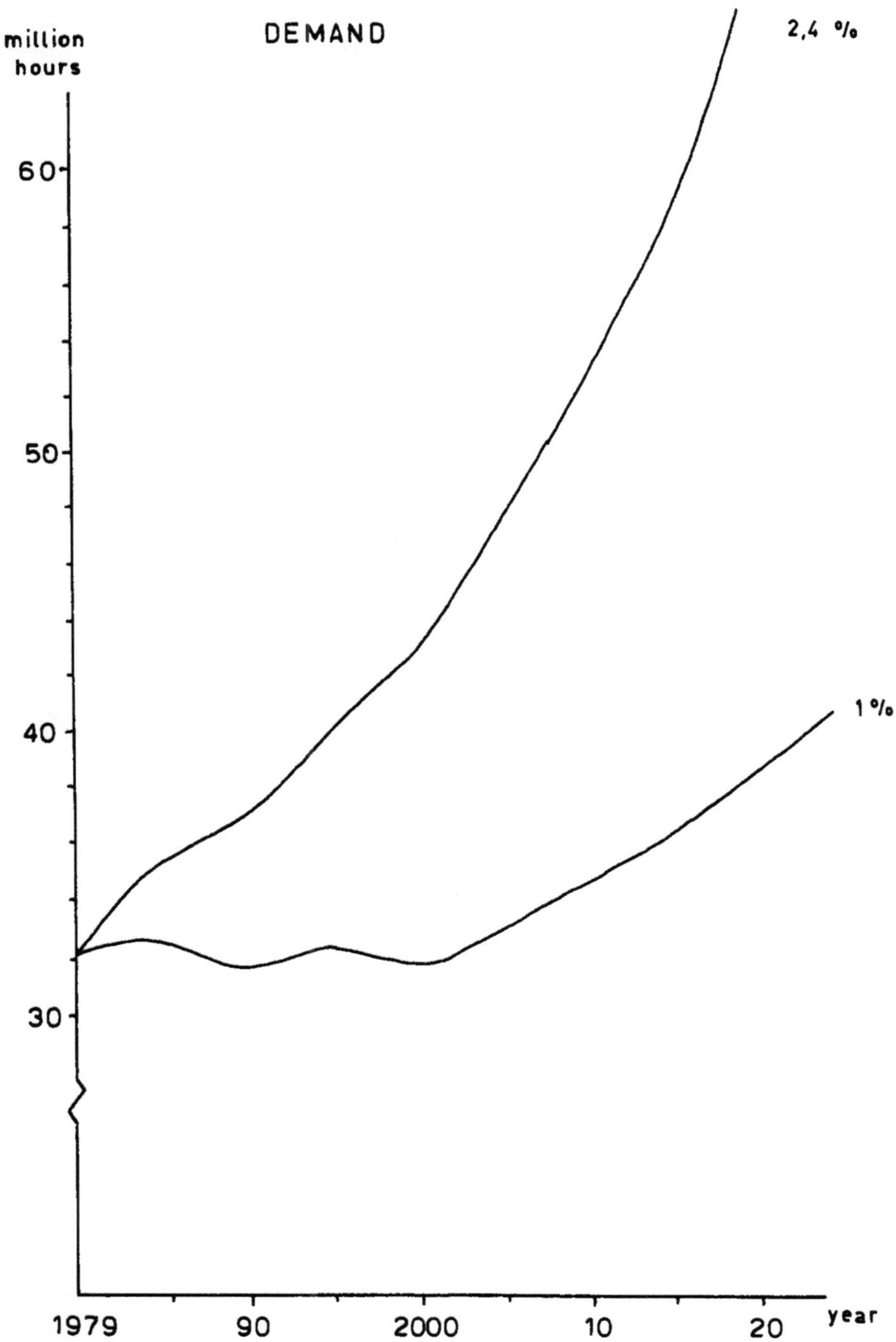

Figure 2

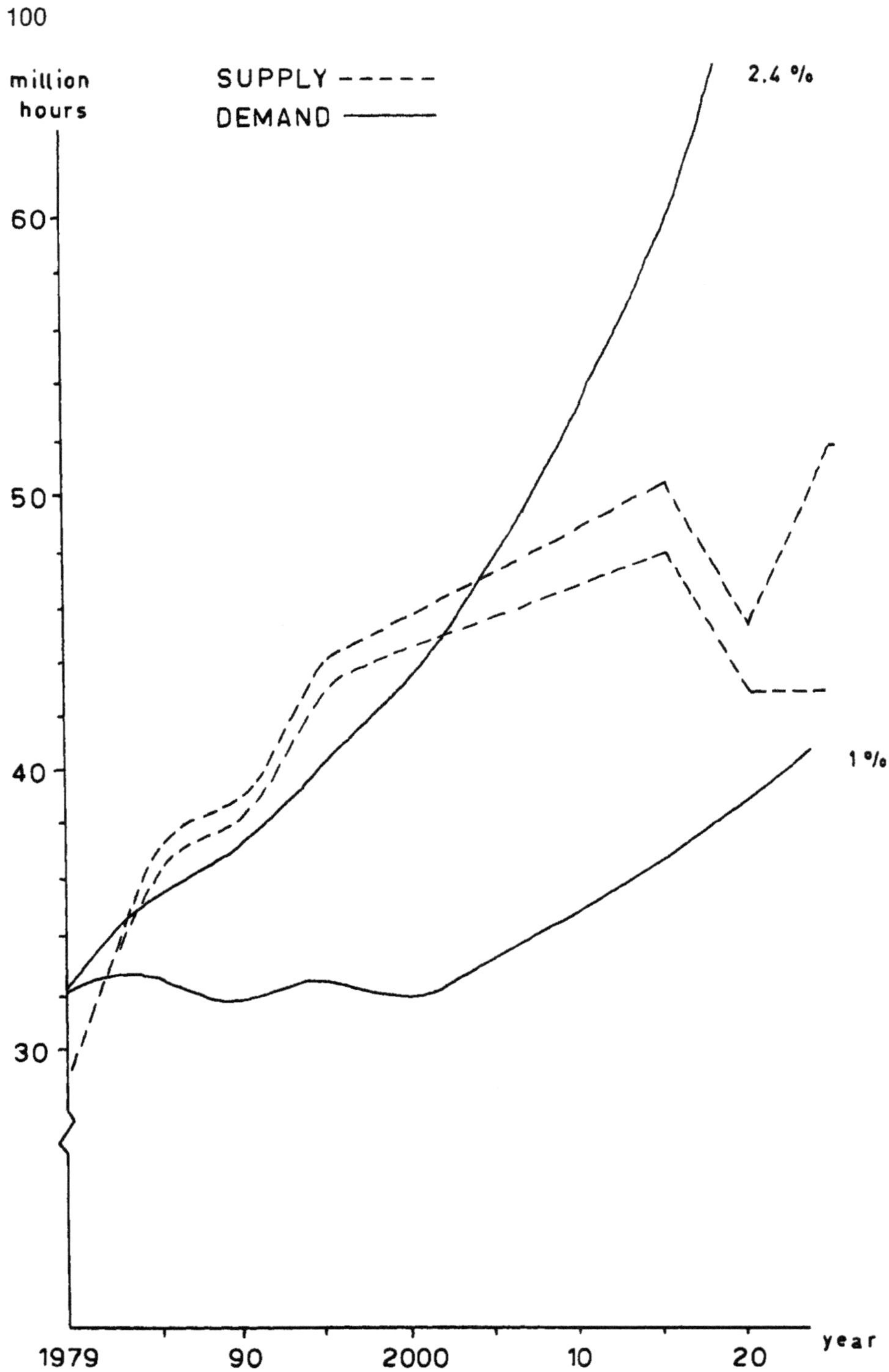
100
million hours
SUPPLY
DEMAND
2.4 %
60
50
40
30
1 %
1979
90
2000
10
20
year

Figure 3

Abrams: at the moment although more male doctors would like to work part-time, it appears that all part-timers, both male and female are now working longer hours, almost full-time.
Milton: in Sweden 97% of the female doctors work full-time, against 92%-95% of other women. In Sweden, full-time means 40 hours a week. In Sweden male-doctors can take children-leave as well as female-doctors can.
Van der Lugt: does Greep have figures on Dutch doctors migrating for the developing countries, and for the USA, Canada, etc.?
Greep: there are about 400 in these sectors. About 250 Dutch doctors in Africa who will come back onto the national market in 3 or 4 years time. The USA has made entry very difficult. The situation in Africa and the Middle-East is changing rapidly with the growth of local medical faculties.
A Danish doctor: the number of working hours per week is extremely important. For instance, in Denmark the junior doctors have reduced their hours, causing a 40% increase in the number employed.

SESSION III:

METHODS AND STRATEGIES IN MANPOWER PLANNING

Health Manpower Planning in Industrialized Countries

B. Eklundh, Ph. D.

The new role of health care

On a recent travel to one of the highly industrialized countries in the European region I tried to get information on the actual situation and foreseen development regarding health manpower. I got different answers which in all indicated that there seemed to be an imbalance between demand and supply of manpower. I was faced with all those expressions that any health manpower planner is familiar with: oversupply, overspecialization, maldistribution and malutilization. Some of the answers stated that there already now seemed to be too much manpower if looking strictly out of a quantitative perspective. On the other hand, if making a qualitative analysis, trying to figure out the real need of health care of the population and the needs for the implementation of the concept 'Health for all by the year 2000' I was told that there was a lack of health manpower with adequate professional competence. On the whole this is a contradictive situation that mainly industrialized countries are facing.

Most systems for the delivery of health care in Europe are in a stage of reorientation and restructuring. The main objective of this process is to provide communities not only with medical care, but also with mechanisms for the prevention of illness and promotion of health. Furthermore, the organization and content of health care has to a much higher extent to be related to the health and social needs of communities.

WHO is strongly supporting this reorientation and has developed a comprehensive policy in that respect known as 'Health for all by the year 2000', which already has been referred to. There are growing demands on health care systems providing new services: expansion of primary health care, of the concept of preventive medicine, promotion of the teamwork approach, and expansion of certain sectors such as mental health, care of the elderly, rehabilitation.

The demands for change are concerned with all levels of health care and appear in spite of the financial constraints that the industrialized societies are facing. It goes without saying that the quality of health care and the implementation of any changes of health care is highly dependant on the knowledge, skills and attitudes of health manpower.

Health care systems have so far been fortunate in having the possibility of solving most problems by expansion. One result of this is the rapid expansion of the number of health personnel. In several countries of the European region, up to or more than 75% of the total cost of health care is devoted to health personnel. Expansion will no longer be possible as more and more pressure will be put on the existing system to make priorities within existing resources. Many health systems in Europe are facing a situation with a zero-growth or even a request to diminish the entire health care system, a situation which the private labour market knows only too well.

In this difficult and challenging situation there are a few items to be underlined to demonstrate the complexity and the importance of the health manpower process. These are the items:

1. A comprehensive policy for health manpower development;
2. Communication and collaboration within and between the systems for health care and education of health professions;
3. The proper utilization of existing resources;
4. The development of systems for information.

A comprehensive policy for health manpower development

The situation regarding health manpower in the industrialized countries is difficult to grasp in a comprehensive way. Many of the perceived problems are relative. The situation analysis done very often utilizes expressions as 'oversupply' and 'overproduction' on the one hand and 'maldistribution' and 'malutilization' on the other.

Such expressions are in a sense political as they indicate an opinion and political decisions can change the entire situation over a right.

Such items as for instance 'oversupply' of 'overproduction' ought at first to be seen in relation to the utilization of manpower. That is how tasks are distributed between different categories of personnel or the actual professional competence of existing personnel to meet emerging demands of health services. Another aspect is the distribution of manpower over a country and between different specialities.

There must be a solid basis for the different activities in the field of health manpower development to which all matters connected with the complex problem of demand and supply have to be related. There is a need for the formulation of a comprehensive health manpower policy as an integrated part of the national health care policy. This policy has to be well elaborated and with a political status that is unquestionable and with the aim to support the fulfilment of the objectives of the nation's overall health care policy.

The concept 'comprehensive' is used as health manpower planners ought to exert influence on as many variables as possible, both regarding quality and quantity based on the existing health manpower policy. Systems for health care and education of health professions are very complex and a number of parallel activities on different levels have to be planned, implemented, monitored and evaluated in a constant process.

Communication and collaboration

This leads over to the second item which is that of *communication and collaboration within and between the systems for health care and education for health professions.*

New directions of health care policy of a society lead to demands for changes both of content and organization of training and education. The planning of education and training of health professionals must be made in close collaboration with health care planning. Today, there is in many countries a considerable imbalance between health care planning and educational planning.

Both systems seem to speak different languages, live on their own and sometimes - compete instead of collaborate. Communication and collaboration are terms with a wide range of meanings. Their specific content may differ according to the particular level of relationship between the health services and the educational system.

The matter of communication and collaboration has been analyzed in depth by WHO in a number of different activities. A general finding is the awareness of the problem and that it is fairly well described. What is lacking, however, is a set of sound concepts and strategies which would allow for a relevant progress in communication and collaboration. A prerequisite to the development of such workable mechanisms for change is an insight into the constraints to better cooperation and collaboration in the field of health care and education.

The recommendations for improvement are mainly focused on the development of liaison mechanisms between the different bodies involved in health manpower development. On several occasions proposals have been raised that an improvement of communication and collaboration cannot be achieved unless a national representative body, in which both the health services and the training system are represented, is set up.

This liaison mechanism should include high-level representatives form each key agency involved: policy-makers, administrators, health planners, providers of health care, educators of the health team and researchers. Such a body could promote national understanding and develop guidelines for action aimed at developing a comprehensive plan for health services and manpower training.

For that purpose it is essential to ensure a sound balance between the centralized and decentralized levels within a country in all matters of decision-making and execution.

The improvement of communication and collaboration is not an easy task since health services and training systems have developed a high level of division of labour which has led to the development of peculiar interests within the system as a whole and thus to a lack of consensus on the desirable changes of the services and the educational concepts.

The improvement of communication and collaboration within and between the health services and the health manpower training systems is narrowly linked to the perspectives of development of a system of primary health care in Europe and thus largely depends on a basic change of the concepts of health and disease.

The proper utilization of existing manpower resources

The scope of the process of health manpower development consists of three main parts, namely *planning, production* and *management*.

In a situation with decreasing financial resources and increasing demands there has to be a focus on health manpower management, the goal of which is to optimize the use of health manpower with the objective to determine manpower distribution and productivity standards, patterns of utilization and non-labour inputs.

In the entire process of health manpower it could be stated that the managerial part is something like a neglected child. Still most countries avoid developing a dynamic and comprehensive approach to the managerial process due to the fact that it is difficult and painful to go into the existing structure of health care and health manpower and start a process of change. Much more effort has to be given to the managerial process in the future to make the best use of existing manpower resources to fulfil actual and foreseen needs.

Within health manpower management there is one activity of great importance and that is *continuing education* of health personnel. Over many years WHO has devoted much attention to the promotion of continuing education, a line of development which in the future will be even more important. In comparison with basic education and specialist or postgraduate training, continuing education is the only instrument to achieve rapid changes or improvements of knowledge, skills and attitudes. With continuing education it is possible to reach health manpower at any time during their professional career. Continuing education is an instrument for change supporting the fulfilment of the objectives of the health care policy and is thus a responsibility not only for individual professionals but also for the entire health care system.

The development of a proper system for information

Decisionmaking in the process of health manpower development is difficult. To avoid uncertainty as much as possible it is vital to have a good system for statistical information for the purpose of monitoring and evaluation. Far too many decisions are based upon limited or obsolete data or knowledge out of personal experience, a kind of anecdotal information. Most countries have, however, systems for statistical information on health manpower but far too often those systems seem to be badly utilized or not adapted to fulfil relevant needs. The system for statistical information must be put into a proper context and its development must be directed in line with the health manpower policy.

WHO activities to promote the health manpower planning

Within the years to come WHO will pay increasing attention to the promotion of the health manpower process. As part of the process of reorientation of health care, it is important for WHO to provide assistance to Member States in the adaptation of the health manpower planning process to the needs of communities and health care systems. The WHO Regional Office for Europe is just now starting a study on Health Services/Manpower Development.

The main aim of the Study is to review the actual situation in Member States in health manpower development and to analyze the methodologies used. The Study will take into account the existing relationship between health services planning and health manpower planning and existing or planned national strategies in the field of health to facilitate and stimulate the process of reorientation. The development towards primary health care, preventive medicine, multiprofessional teamwork, together with the increasing economical constraints, underlines the need for a well functioning system for health manpower planning which, until now, has focused too much on quantitative aspects.

The data collected will be published and circulated to Member States and will form the basis for the future elaboration of guidelines for health manpower planning adapted to the needs of European Member States. With this study and other related activities, such as international and national training activities in health manpower planning, WHO wants to stimulate Member States to the development of coordinated and relevant health manpower planning and rational use of health personnel in order to meet the changing needs of health care systems.

Concluding remarks.

1. The further development of health manpower has to be closely integrated with the health services development.
2. There is a need to formulate, as part of this development, a well-elaborated comprehensive health manpower policy on which there is a national consensus.
3. The concept of communication and collaboration within and between the systems for health care and education of health professions needs attention in order to coordinate the activities of all different bodies involved in the health manpower process.
4. The proper utilization of the existing health manpower resources has to be promoted as part of the managerial process of which continuing education is an important instrument for change.
5. One prerequisite for the proper development of health manpower is a well-functioning statistical information system.
6. WHO is supporting the health manpower development process as it is the basis for achieving reoriented health care systems towards the concept of 'Health for All by the Year 2000'.

Discussion:

Petit: talking about financial constraints in the industrial countries is relative; for instance, from the Tanzanian viewpoint Europe of course is still very rich.
Eklundh: agreed. He emphasized the contradiction in almost all industrial countries, facing financial constraints while there is an oversupply of doctors. However, the ample resources are not adapted to the new demands of the health care system with preventative medicine and primary care.

References

1. Hall, Mejia: Health Manpower Planning: principles, methods, issues. WHO, Geneva, 1978.
2. Hornley, Ray, Shipp, Hall: Guidelines for Health Manpower Planning. WHO, Geneva, 1978.
3. Health Manpower Planning. Report on a workshop, Copenhagen, 19-21 October 1981. WHO Regional Office for Europe, Copenhagen, 1982 (ICP/MPM 028).
4. Relevance of Educational Planning to Health Problems. Report of a Working Group, Kuopio, 1975. WHO Regional Office for Europe, Copenhagen, 1876 (ICP/HMD 008).
5. Country Health Programming as a Determinant of Health Manpower Development Policies. Report of a Working Group, Bern, 1977. WHO Regional Office for Europe, Copenhagen, 1979 (ICP/HMD 056).
6. Global Strategy for Health for All by the Year 2000. WHO, Geneva, 1981.
7. Managerial Process for National Health Development, Guiding Principles. WHO, Geneva, 1981.

Planning of Medical Manpower for Health Care in the Light of a Changing Employment Market

R.M. Lapré, Ph.D.

Introduction

In this paper the analysis of the labour market and the related economical questions will be emphasized. I will not stop at the analysis but I will also make suggestions for an actual policy.

Some problems will occur here since policy making is an activity which should fit the specific situation of a country. Health manpower planning as a systematic preparation for a policy is no exception. Planning, legislation, societal ideas, economic situation, status of the health care workers, etc., vary from country to country.

Because this is an international symposium I will keep the analysis and the policy suggestions somewhat general.

Those aspects which can be generalized will get more attention than any specific aspects. There is yet another restriction. Although the title of the symposium is *Health Manpower Planning*, this gives an undesirable vagueness when all health care workers would be considered undiscriminately and in one breath. For the problems with regard to, for instance, nurses, hospital directors and doctors are completely different, although they are interconnected. Although much of what I am going to say is related to the labour market in health care in general, I will address myself in particular to doctors. I don't do this because I regard doctors as the 'prototype' of the health care worker but for sheer practical reasons. For that matter, it strikes me that in none of the titles of the papers in this programme, medical manpower is mentioned. In the introduction of the preliminary programme however, the 'growing imbalance between the supply and the demand of *medical* manpower' is indicated. Nevertheless, I want to point out, that it would be a dangerous simplification if medical manpower and health manpower were to be regarded as synonyms and if an attempt were made to solve the problem of *health* manpower restricted oneself to the domain of medical manpower. (4, 7, 9, 21 and 22)

In this paper I will focus on some characteristics of the labour market for doctors and on some specific developments in that market: I will discuss the development regarding employment in the light of the socio-economic situation. Arguments will be given that the present restriction of financial resources calls for a stronger regulation of the labour market, which will become evident, among other things, in diminishing possibilities to enter the labour market. Following this line, attention will be given from an economic point of view, to the regulations of the training capacity in order to prevent frictions between the absorption possibilities of the labour market and the supply of doctors. Finally I will go into the income policy to be adopted in the light of the developments in the labour market, and into government influence on this market.

TOPICS

- labour market for physicians
  - characteristics
  - trends
- limitation of financial possibilities
- regulations by government
- entry to the labour market
- regulation of training capacity
- income policy

Figure 1

But first some introductory remarks about the general labour market (10 and 34), for this cannot be seen separately from the labour market for doctors. The predominating problem on the general labour market is diminishing employment, causing an alarming high unemployment. In the countries of the European Community this is currently between 7% (Western Germany) and 14% (Great Britain). Future developments moreover are extremely uncertain. For these depend also on external factors, such as other countries, energy prices, rate of interest, international competition, and these are difficult to control. Furthermore there appear to be practical limits to fully man-made social systems such as health care within desired limits of time.

Generally accepted goals for attacking huge problems such as growing unemployment are also lacking. This accounts for a wavering, ambiguous and discontinuous policy. It is of great consequence for the employment in health care whether the general policy is aimed at the creation of employment in the collective non-profit public sector, or whether the emphasis is placed on stimulation of the private sector. Often a 'slalom' may be observed between these two policy options.

The ambiguity is furthermore promoted by the lack of any adequate policy instrument for realizing a desired policy, within a certain limit of time, or, the instruments being available, by the lack of courage and the incapacity for implementing these. For all these reasons it is not surprising then that the results of planning efforts in many countries have appeared to be very disappointing up till now.(29 and 30)

Some characteristics

A striking characteristic of the labour market for doctors is the extreme professional differentiation, resulting mainly from the differentiation in care processes. Thus we know already of 35 medical specializations in The Netherlands, and there are countries where this number is even higher. Health care has become so complex on account of differentiation and the increase in scale which this involves, that a new caste of managers, sub-managers, planners, information experts, etc., is emerging in order to safeguard cohesion and continuity of the processes. The professional differentiation has already effected the labour market. Some of the consequences are loss of flexibility and an income stimulating effect. Specialization calls for additional years of medical training and leads to monopolies of knowledge. These are the factors that in our Western society lead to income demands and to the social legitimation of a higher income.

This professional differentiation has made it impossible to talk of 'the' labour market for doctors. There exists in fact a labour market per category. The circumstances in each category may be largely similar but often there are essential differences, which makes the position of the interested party on the labour market completely specific. Thus there are, as regards medical professions, considerable differences between the labour market for pediatricians, radiologists, cardiac surgeons, geriatrists, occupational health physicians, psychiatrists, etc., also leading to considerable differences between current employment, future possibilities, work situation, status and income.

Another striking element of the labour market for doctors is the large autonomy in professional practice. There exists a great deal of freedom in choosing methods of curing and caring. It is the doctor who to a great extent determines what should be done, when, by whom and for how long. In other words, it is also the doctor who will influence the demand for health care and thus the demand for supply of physicians. In this respect doctors are able to influence to a large extent their own employment and that of other professions in health care (for instance nurses, para-medical and laboratory personnel). (5) Moreover, the effects of their work are not readily measurable, and an objective judgement from which the redundancy of certain parts of cure and care would become apparent, is extremely difficult. For this reason a surplus of doctors will not become apparent soon. The doctor creates his own production level and since its financing has been safeguarded by legislation in the public sector, there is in principle no obstacle to an unbridled spiralling of growth in demand and supply (20), and not in the last place, of costs.

In relation to the above it should not surprise that the position of doctors on the labour market still is strong. This becomes evident, among other things, in the relatively high incomes. In most Western countries doctors' income are in the highest income bracket. Apart from this, from the immaterial benefits in status and from autonomy of working methods, the profession has a strong appeal. This stimulates the supply of doctors on the labour market.

CHARACTERISTICS OF LABOUR MARKET FOR PHYSICIANS
- - professional differentiation
- - increase of scale
- - monopolies of knowledge
- - autonomy in professional practice
- - high income

Figure 2

Dynamics of the labour market

The labour market for doctors changes continuously. A development which has become more and more obvious in the last years is a stronger restriction in the possibilities for a free choice for work and working conditions. Regulation has increased considerably and in many work situations of doctors hierarchical conditions have developed. (37) Such developments restrict the doctor in his elbow- room to influence the labour market from his microsituation. It is to be expected that these developments will continue. The increasing complexity of health care and the need for cooperation, the growing social control, the demands which are made for integration and cohesion of care, even in relation to facilities outside health care, considerations of equity, but certainly also economical considerations, seem all to provide strong arguments for this.

A strong growth of employment is part of the dynamics of the labour market. This may have been in nearly all Western countries during the last couple of years. Economically three factors have played a part:

1. The relatively high income elasticity: an increase in prosperity causing an even greater increase of demand for health care;
2. The relatively low, or even lack of rise in productivity in health care (3); therefore a greater demand should nearly always lead to an extension of manpower and thus to higher costs;
3. The low price elasticity, which means that a rise in the price of anyone benefit is of little or no influence on the demand for that benefit.

These three factors are mutually re-inforcing in their effect on the increase of employment. This effect should be taken into account in the estimates of future needs. At a declining economic situation the positive effect of the income elasticity will disappear. The demand for those parts of care which are perceived by the public as a certain luxury will then decline even more. Furthermore at a declining economic situation, mechanisms will come into operation causing the price elasticity to rise, for the collective financing of health care will then come under pressure. A need may arise to shift financial responsibility for the costs of health care towards private citizens. In that case expenditures for health care are competing with other expenditures which press on the dwindling private income. In such a situation a price increase will soon lead to a decrease in demand and thus to less employment. In addition the lack of, or at best, the relatively low rise in labour productivity in health care accounts for the fact that this care cannot escape relatively steep price increases. I conclude from that the above factors, which at a growing economy in a process of mutual re-inforcement have led to a considerable increase of employment in health care, will have a cumulative adverse effect at a slackening economy. At a continuing stagnation there is little doubt that there will be a loss of jobs in health care.

DYNAMICS OF THE LABOUR MARKET

in past: cumulative effect of:

- high income elasticity
- lack of rise in productivity
- low price elasticity

Figure 3

Government regulations.

Government plays an important role on the labour market. In Western countries there are various levels of government interference with health care. Although the governments of most Western countries have been rather reserved up till now to directly interfere with the level of employment, the policy they adopt with regard to health care has indeed repercussions on that labour market. It is my impression that when unemployment had not yet risen so dramatically, government interference was mainly aimed at pushing back the rising unemployment. Since this effort has not been very successful, it seems that more emphasis is put on distribution of the (remaining) employment. (11, 12, 18 and 35)

Employment in health care is determined in part by government policy, but up till now mostly in an indirect way, i.e. a policy which promotes the access to benefits, stimulates the demand and gives an incentive to a growth in employment. An increase in the amount of collective resources available for health care will also promote employment. When standards based on legislation or other formal grounds are laid down for the numbers of health care workers of various categories, already a more direct interference with employment occurs. Such standards are known of in many countries. In general they do not yet apply to privately working doctors, but this seems only a matter of time.

This seems likely since in a health care system with restricted financial means any possibilities for an optimal allocation of the various benefits, and in consequence of categories of workers, must be attempted. Government then comes explicitly in a distributive role: employment is distributed. In such a situation, in which the volume of most benefits has been normated, it is not logical that an exception is made for the medical profession, for this would undermine the system. With restricted financial resources it should be prevented that certain benefits attract means at the cost of benefits that have been regulated. In a financially restricted situation planning and setting of priorities are necessary instruments for a public health policy. Both will lead to a restriction of the free entry of doctors to the labour market, should this not yet have been the case. In a situation of regulation the entry may be judged from the point of view of both the available means and the priorities set. The number of doctors to be admitted to the labour market, may then be regarded in connection with the admittance of other workers such as nurses, paramedical, administrative/ technical personnel, etc.

Entry to the labour market

For employed doctors there is per definition no free entry. They will only be able to work professionally when a job is available. For doctors working privately as free entrepreneurs, this used to be different. (17) Free entry in most cases means also the possibility of rendering services to a self-desired extent, which has in general led to a relatively high income. The medical certificate thus opened the door to the labour market, whereas the individual position on the market could be manipulated thereafter by influencing the demand. The absorption power of the labour market in health care has decreased on account of the current lack of financial resources. When medical schools continue to train more doctors than the sector is able to adsorb, a barrier for entry is unavoidable. This calls for more regulations and more government interference.

There is an interaction between the need for regulation of the entry to the labour market and the size of the training capacity. The better the latter is tuned to the absorption capacity of the labour market, the less need for a regulation of access. Consequently here lies a clearcut policy option.

The medical schools cannot be expected to curtail their training capacity on their own accord, on account of labour market considerations. Even in countries where the minister of Public Health is (partly) responsible for the training capacity for doctors, such an adjustment appears to be mostly lacking. (25)

Limiting access also has its drawbacks. Care should be taken that not a government-limited 'closed shop' situation should be created, i.e. a situation of high-salaried privileged doctors who won't have to fear competition from others, once they have been permitted access. (13)

GOVERNMENT INFLUENCE ON LABOUR MARKET

- indirect: financial policy, health care policy
- direct (distributive role): norms for numbers of personnel

Figure 4

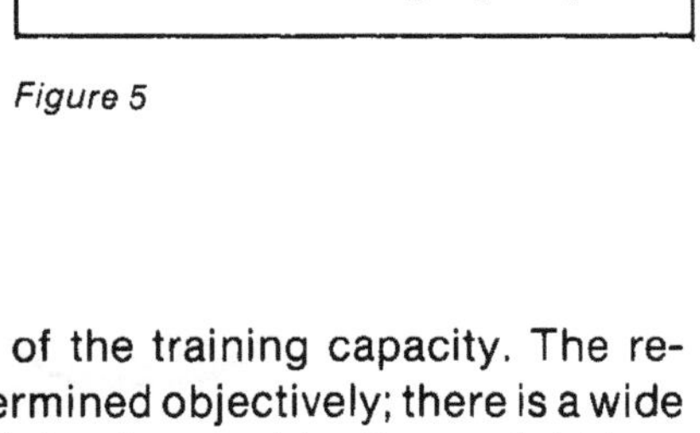

Figure 5

Regulation of training capacity

Many problems attach to a regulation of the training capacity. The requirements in health care cannot be determined objectively; there is a wide margin in which benefits are mutually interchangeable; the social ideas about what is desirable are subject to changes; there are permutations in policy, all of which may have important consequences for the training capacity. (2, 8, 26, 30 and 32) Estimates often prove to be wrong in practice.

Ray and Andreano remark in this context, 'nearly all the manpower forecasting, whether in developing of developed countries, restricted sectorally or covering all occupations, has proved to be a failure'. (29, p.288)

Communicating vessels

The main part of the financial means earmarked for health care, about 65% to 75%, is spent on costs to bring in labour. These costs consist of two components; a volume component consisting of the number of persons employed, and a price component, consisting notably of their incomes. In the metaphor of the communicating vessels it becomes clear that when we take as point of departure a certain amount of financial resources, both the total amount of resources to be spent and the incomes are important policy options. The total amount of liquid symbolizes the available amount of financial means. The number of doctors to be employed and the height of the income of the doctors are indicated, each by the level in one of the two communicating vessels. When the financial resources which society wishes to spend on health care are increasing, both the number of doctors and the income may go up; the level in both vessels increases. When the level in the vessel, showing the income, is kept at the same height, or is being reduced, the level in the other vessel (the number of doctors) may go up more.

Health care has been brought into the public sector even more. The determination of the financial resources earmarked to that goal, is a process of social consideration and of politics. The appropriateness of the policy options will not be discussed within this context. This is not relevant to the discussion and should be regarded as given data. In view of the precarious economic situation it is very likely that the public expenditures for health care will come under pressure even further.

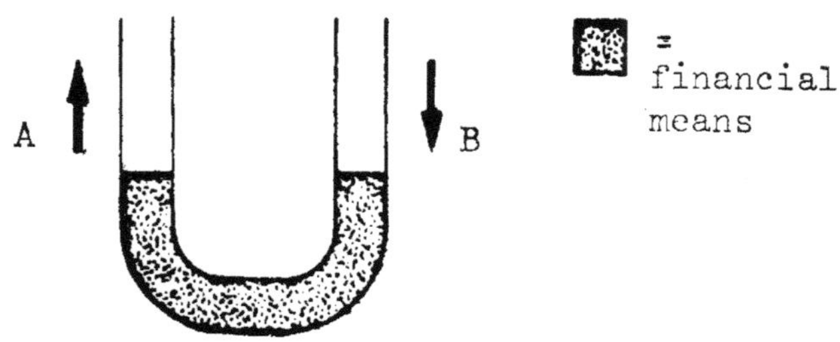

A = amount of doctors

B = income of doctors

Figure 6

Apart from this it can be established that, notably in countries where the health care is not financed out of taxation, a change in approach is taking place, or (recently) has taken place. Roughly the model changes as follows. It was:

number of doctors multiplied by income results in costs, and costs have as outcome available financial resources.

Now this model has changed into:

available resources result in a certain number of doctors with a certain income.

In all the factors of the first model there occur largely autonomous developments which cannot be influenced. The costs and the available financial resources are a resultant of the number of doctors and costs of doctors' services. In the second model the point of departure is the restricted budget. The total expenditures and thus the factors causing these expenditures, should here be turned to the restricted budget. This means then the number of doctors and their incomes.

POINT OF DEPARTURE

was: doctors x income = costs

→ available financial resources

should be: available resources

→ doctors x income

Figure 7

Income policy

Relative scarcity is reflected in income as cost of the production factor labour: relatively high incomes give an indication as to the presence of scarcity on the labour market. The steep increase of the number of doctors of the last decades has not led to surplusses until recently. This came about because the demand expanded likewise, and so did the means for financing the higher costs. The relative scarcity was thus maintained. With their growing influx young doctors could more or less automatically create their own jobs. Now that the number of jobs is going to be regulated in conformity with the existing macro-economic limits, the disappearing scarcity of doctors may become manifest and surplusses may become obvious. In principle an income-reducing effect will develop out of these new labour conditions. Such an effect has the advantage that the restricted financial resources may be distributed among more medical manpower. The employment of doctors is thus promoted. The line of thought then is:

The scarcity has disappeared, consequently the doctors' incomes should be brought to a 'normal level', but this is not yet the case. (36) What is normal depends, among other things, on social circumstances in any country. In The Netherlands the so-called norm income should be wielded, an income level which corresponds with that of the highest salary scales in government service.

One should realize that restriction of the supply of young doctors, as a result of which there will be no surplusses, should not lead to an income policy based on a scarcity of doctors. A policy for a restricted supply should be conducted simultaneously with an income policy. Of course restriction of supply should not again lead to scarcity and income stimulating effects. Since health care has developed into an integral part of the Western welfare state and since the financial resources largely are provided collectively, it is society also that has the right to decide and will have to decide, on the supply of new doctors, on the access to the labour market, and on the income that is gained from the collective financial means.

INCOME POLICY

to be based on the fact
that scarcity of physicians'
services has disappeared

Figure 8

Recommendation

I want to conclude this paper with the recommendation to work on a proposal for a practical approach to tune the training capacity for the various categories of medical professionals to the size of the health care sector determined by society. A process should be started by which tiny but definite steps forward should be valued more than broad fundamental theoretical considerations. The problem does not lie in the first place within the technical realm of the scientific method of manpower planning, but in the political will and the extent of social consensus. A policy should be developed for obtaining this measure of social consensus. Moreover the still lacking instruments for implementing this manpower policy (legislation, financial measurements, information, consultation procedures), should be provided for. I hope this symposium will lead to more than a beautiful book of proceedings. Words alone will not suffice for a health manpower policy that has the courage to go against vested interests and traditional views.

RECOMMENDATIONS

- tune training capacity to societal demand
- start a political process of achieving consensus
- develop the necessary instruments for implementation of objectives
- apply a practical and incremental approach

Figure 9

Discussion:

Vrijland, chairman: reminded that the income of a specialist is only part of the total costs engendered by him.
Lapré: agreed. It is certain that the specialist has a much greater effect on costs than his income alone.
Someone from the audience: asked Lapré to restate his argument against restricting entry to training in favour of introducing an income policy.
Lapré: if you restrict income per doctor, for a given amount of money, you can employ more doctors, and thus you don't have to restrict entry.
Brearley: when doctors were in short supply, they could command a high income. The situation has changed. Does Lapré think that doctors should be preferentally rewarded to compensate for the long period of study?
Lapré: said that there are other groups who have also long study periods. Secondly health care is not a classical free-market situation. Fees are agreed upon by collective bargaining. When you regulate some parts of the system, it is very difficult to leave other parts free. By budgetary restriction, the restricted salaries tend to be penalized while the free-market ones remain untouched.
Vrijland, chairman: invited one of the representatives of the Dutch Association of Specialists to comment on this but got no reply.

Vissers: the speaker did not mention incentives for the specialist for instance to provide quality or cost-effectiviness. In Holland the clinician himself defines what should be done in a particular case and thus makes it difficult for somebody else to regulate his work. You have to build in positive incentives.
Lapré: quality is very difficult to measure, so when starting planning it is better to take other (measurable) entities into consideration.
Vissers: said that legislation on quality is difficult, the specialist will have an alternative view on this to the legislation.
Lapré: didn't agree that the legislator has to define quality: it is better to plan on the existing situation.

References:

1. N. de Boer en F.R. Veeneklaas. Het arbeidsaanbod op lange termijn. E.S.B., 15-11-1978, pag. 1160-1164.
2. B.S. Bloom, O.L. Peterson. Physician manpower expansionism: a policy revies. Annals of International Medicine. Vol. 90, no. 2, Febr. 1979, pag. 249-256.
3. Centraal Planbureau. Macro-economische verkenning 1982. 's-Gravenhage, 1981.
4. Council Working Party. Medical manpower, staffing and training requirements. British Medical Journal, 19 May 1979, pag. 1365-1376.
5. Department of Health and Social Security. Medical Manpower - The next twenty years. A discussion paper. H.M.S.O., London, 1979.
6. S.R. Engleman. External economic influences on N.H.S. manpower. In Mac. Lachlan, Stocking and Shegog ed., pag. 169-183.
7. J. Fahs, T. Choi, K. Barchas, P. Zakariasen. Indicators of need for health care personnel: the concept of need, alternative measures employed to determine need, and a suggested model.
8. T.L. Hall. Demand. In Hall en Mejia, 1978, pag. 57-89.
9. T.L. Hall, A. Mejia. Editors. Health manpower planning. Principles, methods, issues. W.H.O., Geneva, 1978.
10. F. van den Heuvel. Sectorale werkgelegenheidsontwikkelingen en werkgelegenheidsbeleid in Nederland. Intermediair, 15 aug. 1980, pag. 49-55.
11. F. van den Heuvel en J.J. Siegers. Sectorale werkgelegenheidsontwikkelingen en sectorstructuurbeleid in Nederland. Sociaal Maandblad Arbeid, febr.1980.
12. J.J. van Hoof, A.J. Mantel en M.A. van der Woude. De toekomst van de arbeidsmarkt en het arbeidsmarktbeleid van de toekomst.
13. D. van Ingen. Toelatingsbeleid hoger onderwijs. E.S.B., 9-12-1981, pag. 1226-1229.
14. J.A. van Kemenade. Nota hoger onderwijs in de toekomst. Tweede Kamer, Zitting 1975-1976, 13.733, nos. 1-2.
15. R. Klein. Policy options for medical manpower. British Medical Journal, 9 July 1977, pag. 136-137.
16. D. Lahaye. Numerus Clausus . . . ook in België. Redactioneel. Tijdschrift Soc. Geneesk., 59, no. 4, 1981, pag. 101.
17. Land. Spec. Ver. Vestigingsbeleid en manpower planning Utrecht, 1980.
18. P.A.G. Lansbergen. Werkgelegenheid en collectieve sector. Intermediair, 25 jan. 1980, pag. 15-23.
19. R.M. Lapré. Financiële begrenzingen in de gezondheidszorg. In: Gezondheidszorg onder druk. Ph. Idenburg, G.A. de Jong, J.P. Kasdorp, R.M. Lapré. Samson, Alphen a/d Rijn, 1982.

20. R.M. Lapré. Vraag en aanbod medische specialisten. Medisch Contact. jrg. 35, no. 48, 28 november 1980, pag. 1487-1490.
21. G.Mc. Lachlan, B. Stocking and R. Shegog. Editors. Patterns for uncertainty-Planning for the greater medical profession. The Nuffield Provincial Hospitals Trust. 1979.
22. M. Lynch. The physician 'shortage': the economists' mirror. The Annals of the American Academy of political and social science. Feb. 1972.
23. A. Maunard and A. Walker. Doctor manpower 1975-2000. Alternative forecasts and their resource implications. Report for the Royal Commission on the Health Service. H.M.S.O., London, April 1978.
24. A. Mejia, T. Fülöp. Health manpower planning: an overview. In Hall and Mejia, pag. 9-30.
25. A. Majia, H. Pizurki, E. Rayston. Physician and nurse migration. Analysis and plicy implications. W.H.O., Geneva, 1979.
26. D.R. Mc.Nutt. G.M.E.N.A.C.: Its manpower forecasting framework. A.J.P.H., (Ver. Staten), 71, 10, Oct. 1981, pag. 1116-1123.
27. H. Nys. De toegang tot de medische opleiding in de verzorgingsstaat. Acta Hospitalia 1978, no. 4, pag. 358-388.
28. J. Pool. Instroombeperking schijnoplossing? Medisch Contact, no. 17, 24 april 1981, pag. 501-504.
29. D. Ray, R. Andreano. Economics of health manpower planning. In Hall and Mejia, 1979, pag. 277-298.
30. D.J. Schneider, R. Bilgard. A prospective for health manpower planning. Health Services Report. Vol. 87, no. 5, May 1972, pag. 399-405.
31. H.V. Stambler. Health manpower for the nation. A look ahead at the supply and the requirements. Public Health Reports, 94, Jan./Febr. 1979, pag. 3-10.
32. J.D. Stockle, R. Goldstein. Views from the clinic: doctors, jobs and money in the U.S.A. Editorial comment. Soc. Sci. and Med. 14A, 1980, pag. 89-90.
33. H.R. Verwers. Naar 24.000 specialisten in het jaar 2000. Over norminkomen en normdagtaak. Medisch Contact, no. 40, 2 oktober 1981.
34. A.M.C. Vissers. Werkgelegenheid, werkloosheid en arbeidsmarktgedrag in de jaren '80. Sociaal Maandblad Arbeid, maart 1981.
35. W. van Voorden. Op het grensval van arbeidsverhoudingen en arbeidsmarkt. E.S.B., 8 oktober 1980.
36. Werkgroep Inventarisatie Inkomens Medische Beroepen. Ontwikkelingen op de arbeidsmarkt voor artsen. Medisch Contact, no. 38, 19 sept. 1980, pag. 1155-1157.
37. Wetenschappelijke Raad voor het Regeringsbeleid. Vernieuwingen in het arbeidsbestel. Staatsuitgeverij, 's-Gravenhage, 1981.
38. W.H.O. Guidelines for health manpowerplanning. P. Hornby, D. Ray, P. Shipp and T. Hall. Geneva, 1980.
39. A. Wildafski. If planning is everything, maybe it's nothing. Policy Sciences, 4 (1973) pp. 127-153.

Consequences of Manpower Planning for the Educational Systems in Europe

Brearley, M.S., F.R.C.S.

At the time of signing the Medical Directives on Mutual Recognition of Doctors qualifying diplomas and the coordination of their training (1) (16th June, 1975), the Council of Ministers also issued a Decision setting up an Advisory Committee on Medical Training (ACMT). (2 and 3) The task of this committee as defined in its terms of reference is to ensure 'a comparably demanding standard of medical training in the Community, with regard both to basic training and further training'. In practice the committee has sought to foster not only comparably high but also continuously improving standards. In doing so it has repeatedly found itself confronted with manpower problems and the questions concern not only the Consequences of Manpower Planning for the Educational Systems in Europe which is the title of this paper but also the reciprocal matter of the Consequences of Educational Needs for Manpower Planning.

I now propose to present simple concrete issues which have emerged and some of the conclusions to which they point.

If there is a single conclusion encompassing all the rest, it is that in medical education quality requires manpower planning and where this is lacking, its absence is the greatest single cause of educational insufficiency.

For junior doctors, most of whom have but recently completed basic undergraduate training, are now personally engaged in specialist training and have still to find the employment which will constitute their future professional career, the inter-relation of Manpower Planning and Education is crucial. Within it are embraced the future quality of medical practice and the future prospects of young doctors.

Both at basic and specialist level, the ACMT found itself straight away up against the problem of the educational consequences excessive numbers uncontrolled by any plan.

The economic and personal consequences do not fall within the purview of the ACMT but in strictly educational terms the absence of a properly determined relationship between the numbers of trainees and the educational resources available for their training has proved to be one of the most obstinately recurring difficulties militating against quality in training. There are three operative factors which must be brought into balance; number of trainees, quality of training and resources required; and four possible strategies of all of which examples can be cited:

1. limitation of number to allow optimal training with available resources;
2. expansion of resources to allow optimal training of whatever number present themselves;
3. acceptance of whatever standard may be possible with available resources and unplanned numbers;
4. determination of numbers in relation to medical manpower needs and consequential determination of educational resources to provide optimal training for these.

The first three solutions may result in the production of too many or too few fully trained doctors in toto and within the total number; and in the case of specialist training too many in some branches and too few in others. The totally laissez-faire third solution which has existed widely until recent time also incurs the probability of inequality of standards between different countries and between different specialties and is therefore objectionable on educational grounds. The choice between the other possibilities is not determined by educational considerations but by factors appropriately considered in other sessions of this symposium but I would suggest that in the real world of Europe in the 1980's, only the fourth solution bears any relation to the actual needs or likely resources.

Such a policy however can only be carried out if:

1. appropriate manpower planning machinery exists;
2. appropriate machinery exists to select the required number of trainees from those seeking to enter;
3. no legal obstacle exists to prevent such selection.

We have already heard in the previous session how these matters stand in four member states of the European Communities and one non-member. Overall, the position for basic (undergraduate) medical studies as ascertained by the ACMT was that in 1981, three countries (Belgium, Italy and Luxembourg) had no limits and therefore no selection, while Germany, Denmark, France, Ireland, The Netherlands and U.K. had some form of numerus clausus though not always at the point of admission and not necessarily related to estimates of manpower needs and all operated different methods of selection. Indeed the present national laws of some member states utterly prevent any control of university entry based on future manpower needs. This is a situation which may well be defensible in relation to non-vocational studies which may be a prelude to many different careers, especially if the course involves no personal supervision or practical work. For medical studies which lead only to a medical career and which call for a great deal of closely supervised practical clinical and laboratory work, the present demands for enrolment are over-running both the possibilities of effective instruction and future employment. Such laws are an obsolete survival from times and conditions of the past.

Undergraduate Education

Much time has been spent on the ACMT on studies of the content required for a basic (undergraduate) course of good quality which will lead to the status of doctor. They define such a course as 'the entire amount of theoretical and clinical education, leading to the knowledge which should be common to all doctors whatever their future orientation' (4), and then recommend that 'the clinical training given during basic medical training should be so organized as to take account of the fact that most doctors will devote their entire professional lives to the practice of one or other branch of clinical medicine; this training should take up a large part of the study programme and cover the main clinical disciplines and specialized fields; special attention should be paid to general practice; it should be so planned as to lead to a high level of clinical qualification and competence; for example, students should be trained to establish the patient's clinical history, assimilate the facts related by the patient, carry out a complete clinical examination and critically evaluate the results; a substantial part of clinical training should be devoted to simulating, as far as possible, the actual conditions of medical practice; students should be able in small groups to question and examine specific patients and should be given the opportunity to establish a personal relationship with these patients, at least for the duration of an illness; lastly, training should aim to develop suitable professional personal and ethical attitudes in the student, including the ability to appreciate, understand and deal with sensitively the personal as well as the medical problems of his patients; in this respect explicit instruction may help but must be supported by personal experience and the teacher's example'. (5)

Elsewhere, the ACMT point out that the basic training 'provides the only education on matters outside his own specialty which the future specialist is certain to have had. It should therefore be comprehensive, leaving no important areas of total ignorance. Moves to shorten it by omission of all instruction in some diciplines e.g. opthalmology, dermatology or otolaryngology, or their relegation to a list of options of which only some need be studied will lead to the production of specialists who are not fully educated doctors'.(6) Moreover a doctor who qualifies today at the age of 23 may expect to see enormous changes in medical practice in the ensuing four decades of his professional life. Old specialties (including possibly his own) may contract, disappear or become utterly transformed, while entirely new specialties may arise. The basic course must equip him for such a future both by the breadth and depth of its coverage of the basic principles and skills, and by inculcating adaptability, intellectual curiosity and the habit of continuous self-education.

At the present time many basic medical courses do not fulfil the desiderata just outlined. In the ACMT's opinion 'in many medical schools there are too many students undergoing clinical training in relation to the number of teachers and patients' and 'too much emphasis is placed on theoretical teaching . . . at the expense of clinical and practical experience'. (7) The two observations are linked by the fact that it is not difficult to provide an extra course of lectures for a class of several hundred though it may be impossible to teach them all a wide range of clinical skills. The result is likely to be a doctor who knows all about vector cardiography but cannot recognize heart sounds.

Intensive prolonged clinical instruction in small groups and in close contact with patients is highly demanding of manpower and resources and no country is likely under present conditions to feel able to provide it to large numbers of students who are destined not to finish the course or having done so not to be able to find medical work. Economic constraints make the provision of such high quality education feasible only for students of assured quality who also have a reasonably assured prospect of medical employment. The manpower planning and selection process required to achieve this is therefore effectively a precondition of educational quality. Having got student numbers right, a second act of resource and manpower planning must follow in order to make available the right number of teachers, patients, hospital beds, laboratory bench spaces and so forth. In its 'Report & Recommendations concerning the problems of the balance between the number of Medical Students and the resources needed for their Training' (8) the ACMT has studied this problem and noted the 'to increase the resources available to the faculties of medicine for the training of the increased number in students, the following measures have been taken by the Member States: new faculties of medicine have been opened in The Netherlands, Denmark, the United Kingdom, France, Belgium, Germany and Italy.

In Belgium, Denmark, Germany, the United Kingdom, Italy, France and The Netherlands, agreements have been established between the faculties of medicine and the extra-university sectors (non-university hospitals, other organizations and practising doctors) with a view to increasing the scope for practical training.

In each country the number of teachers has been increased, but 'there is some disparity among Member States in the numbers of medical students and the teachers available in the medical faculties'. They go on to recommend a minimum teacher : student ratio of 1 : 10 in preclinical departments and 1 : 5 in clinical ones. (Owing to the great complexity of the situation, involving individuals wholly of only partly employed by the universities and wholly or partly engaged in teaching, these figures are only a broad indication and it is necessary for a better understanding to read the whole report. Equally difficult studies relating to training beds are still in progress.)

Specialist (Postgraduate) Training

In the field of specialist training* the same triangle of forces uniting numbers, resources and quality constitutes the essential core of the problem but, separate assessment and planning are called for specialty by specialty. Moreover, the problems are further complicated by the essentially different nature of specialist training which is not just a course of instruction but a progressive programme of learning by doing.

The medical directive 75/363/EEC laid down the principle of personal participation of the specialist trainee 'in the activity and in the responsibilities of the establishments concerned' and the ACMT's Report and Recommendations on the General Problems of Specialist Training III/D/732/2/78 (III/D/1904/79) goes on to recommend that this should be achieved by carrying out the training in remunerated full-time posts with a service element (with special provision for part-time training). This introduces several new manpower aspects into the situation.

In the first place, the trainee is providing services within the health system and himself constitutes part of its manpower. Secondly in training institutions when, as is frequently the case, there are numbers of trainees, the more senior ones contribute to the training of the more junior ones. Thirdly the need to find training of practical work means that in the larger specialties, the work flow of the university hospitals is not alone sufficient to offer all the posts required and non-university hospitals also need to be utilized. As with the basic training some breadth of outlook is desirable so that the specialist understands related subjects and is also equipped to cope with future changes in his own specialty. Specialties tend to fall into families and training should proceed through a common trunk of related specialties adapted to the needs of the ultimate specialty to which it leads.

The operation of such a system of training involves planning at many levels. It affects the provision of medical services to the public, the staffing of hospitals and similar institutions, the finding of employment for trainees and the ultimate employment of specialists. The arrangements through which these functions are carried out vary widely between countries.

At the same time the bodies determining the content and standard of training which are equally diverse, are concerned with training issues which interact with matters of employment. Training bodies are concerned not only with standards of care and academic facilities, and with the recognition of posts for training but also with questions of hours of work, duty rotas, study leave, rotation of staff and so forth in which a conflict of interests may arise with employing bodies.

At the present time there are still member states of the European Com-

* using the term to include also general practitioner vocational training.

munity which do not have national competent authorities for specialist training, and do not carry out specialist training through paid posts with progressive responsibility. The standard of practical clinical skill attained by specialist trainees is therefore not everywhere of a comparably high standard.

Granted such a diversity of institutions both for health care and for training, no single formula can be recommended but the basic principles remain: specialists should be trained in numbers related to future needs and the quality of their training especially their practical clinical training should be assured by an adequate number of suitable training posts under the close supervision of the training authorities.

In conclusion therefore, I would repeat my opening summary – that in medical education, quality requires manpower planning and that when this is lacking, its absence is the greatest single cause of educational insufficiency. In addition I would suggest that this planning calls for suitable institutions. These are already well developed in some countries and hardly exist in others. In matters of detail there is opportunity for variety but certain principles are inviolable among which I would suggest four:

1. The numbers in training must have rational relationship to career prospects.
2. There must be a satisfactory system of selection.
3. Training resources must be provided such as will allow the highest possible standard of training for the determined number.
4. The institutions required to realize these objectives must give effective power to the organized medical profession including the trainees and to the competent authorities responsible for academic standard as well as to the bodies whoever they may be, responsible for providing the resources and financing the medical work force.

Discussion

Van Egmond: asked whether the speaker agreed that instead of restricting the number of trainees, it would be better to restrict the working hours to give each trainee more study time etc.? How many hours should there be in a trainee's working week?

Brearley: difficult to say: too many hours mean the trainee is too tired to benefit from his experience, too few hours mean too little experience. He said 'On hours I would have thought that, knowing the fact that there are 24 hours in every day, and it is usually considered appropriate to work for 8, play for 8 and sleep for 8, that something like a 5 day, eight hours week would be a suitable starting point for the discussion'.

References

1. 75/362 & 75/363 EEC.
2. 75/364 EEC.
3. CCFM in French.
4. A.C.M.T. Report on General Tendencies in Basic Medical Training III/D/32/1/78 (III/D/1904/79).
5. A.C.M.T. Recommendation on the Clinical Training of Doctors III/D/33/2/78 (III/D/1904/79).
6. A.C.M.T. Report and Recommendations on the General Problem of Specialist Training M/D/732/2/78 (III/D/1904/79).
7. A.C.M.T. Recommendation on the Clinical Training of Doctors III/D/33/1/78 (III/D/1904/79).
8. III/D/230/4/80.

SESSION IV:

APPROACHES TO THE ROLE OF GOVERNMENT IN MANPOWER PLANNING

The Role of Government in Health Manpower Planning in Hungary

I. Forgács, M.D.

Introductory remarks

The health insurancy has been including the whole population since 1975 in Hungary. In this respect the health care is a right of citizenship and free of charge.

The health service as well as the health manpower planning, development, education and organization is governed by the ministry of Health. The supervision is *direct* in the respect of medical universities, of the health college, in some forms of nurse education and in all forms of post-graduate and continuing education. The national institutes belong also directly to the ministry of Health.

About 80% of in-patient and 95% of out-patient services and the PHC, the social care and the larger part of rehabilitation are directed by the local councils but medically supervized by the national institutes and so indirectly by the ministry of Health.

The planning of health service and health manpower is closely connected with the actual five years plans. The planning of health manpower takes place in the ministry of Health according to the following methods:
- situation analysis by different demographical, ill-health, health manpower and other relevant parameters,
- taking into account the possibilities and relations to other sectors,
- aims and objectives according to the needs, demands and supply,
- matching the above mentioned factors, and
- monitoring and evaluation.

Demographical

The basic demographical figures showing the health condition of the population (the average life expectancy at birth time, mortality) have gone through unfavourable changes during the last decade, taking into consideration both their quantity and tendency. The present level of satisfying the needs and the several factors influencing the health condition and needs of the population indicate that there will be a growing tendency in the health needs of the population during the next two decades.

Demographic factors have a permanent differentiative influence on the probable structure of the morbidity and on the use of health institutions. For the year 2000 a fourhundred thousand - decrease in the number of the population is foreseen, which will concern mainly the younger age groups, while the number of those above sixty is going to increase by two hundred thousands. This process of the ageing of the population implies a growth in the coincidence of diseases and the use of institutions (both preventive-curative and social).

Mother, infant and child protection plays an essential role among the objectives of our health policy, aiming at increasing and stabilizing the level of fertility and protecting the health condition of the new generations, which coincides with our long term population policy. During the next period an increase in environmental harms and potential sources of danger is foreseen.

Ill-health Status.

During the next twenty years a fundamental task will be the prevention, therapy, care and rehabilitation first of all of cardiovascular diseases, accidents, tumour diseases and mental diseases. Our long term special programmes for the effective curing of these branches of diseases must be realized in a coordinated, periodically task-oriented, progressive way. The number of the newly discovered cases will be increasing further because of the spreading of preventive medicine, of screening, and of the early discovery of cases previously not known. This slightly increases the number of the so-called first appearences, and a dynamic increase in the regular uses is probable caused by a more frequent practice of care. A reasonable limitation in the number of claims can be achieved only by a more effective endeavour to cure them resultfully and definitively.

The use of in-patient institutes (the proportion of hospitalization) will slightly increase, while the average duration of care can be shortened by a more intensive examination and the widening of the range of treatments in out-patient care. The increase in the use of hospitals can be preserved on an acceptable level only if the conditions of primary health care, screening, social care, are developed in a purposeful and coordinated way.

Care

Care - also as the main method of preventive medicine - must be gradually expanded in a way that it must preserve its tending towards special branches of diseases and special age-groups. Though the whole range care of the population cannot be realized by 2000, it is essential that this kind of activity must be the main territory of primary health care.

The extension of screening must be done with concentration on branches of diseases of national health importance, and with unique methods, optimal periodicity. So the care of selected patients is mainly the task of primary health care. The role and importance of primary health care in the structure of health services will be essentially growing. That is why it has to reform its system of relations with the other branches of health provision. The level of training and post-graduate training of general practitioners must be increased, and the conditions from their work must be secured. We have to work out acceptable methods for improving the interest and work performance of GP's.

The tasks of health and social nursing and care have been presented in a more and more combined way (at the same person, or group, or population) that is why the services of home nursing and the forms of district social care must be developed in a coordinated way, it has to work under the unified special direction of the general practitioner, and the model of the organizational union must be worked out and realized.

In the field of mother, infant and child protection perinatal mortality must and can be further decreased with the improving of the care (perinatal care, infant protection) providing a healthier reproduction. The whole range care of larger - especially urban - child populations must be realized by a better coordinated, complementary and not overlapping function of district and school health provision.

Problems of ageing

One of the main questions of the future is the perspective of the care for the elderly. In the framework of it traditional forms must be developed proportionally (e.g. the number of day-homes for the elderly must be raised to be three times more, and the number of places in social homes with 70%-75%), on the other hand new forms of care must be created and developed, e.g. boarding houses for the elderly, but first of all social care at home. The activity of the society regarding care - besides the present and extendable forms and institutional network of social care - must be tended towards the activation of the population (families, groups, individuals, organizations), as their participation in fulfilling these tasks is essential.

Rehabilitation

Rehabilitation, which is an extremely important task from the point of view of the future society, is practised on the common basis of the network of health and social institutions. The tendency towards the growth in the number of the disabled can be stopped only by building up an overall system of rehabilitation. In the field of medical rehabilitation, within the hospitals the in-patient background of cardiological, locomotor and mental rehabilitation must be developed in organic unity with the out-patient sections. Professional rehabilitation is the key issue in building up the overall rehabilitation system. Rehabilitation is a complex task of social policy, which can be raised to the necessary level only by the planned and coordinated work of all the necessary organs and institutes.

Progressivity

When working out, taking and realizing special-organizational measures, the principles of progressive health care must be asserted. In the spirit of this the practice should be that each patient should get health provision of the level and in the form his disease and condition demands it. Within the integrated in-patient institution, during the course of forming the special internal structure, besides the sections for intensive and active care, sections for long term care must be organized.

The vertical levels of progressive provision (town-county-regional-national) must secure the division of work among the institutes. On the basis of the probable special tasks till 2000 it can be foreseen that the town level can need 60%-70%, the county level 20%-25%, the regional 8%-12%, and the national 2%-3% of all the beds. The different levels must be developed towards the marked tendencies, without taking into consideration the spontaneous organizations and the local prestige interests.

Health manpower

Taking into consideration the demands raised by the development in the network of provision, changes in the structure and qualitative factors, by 2000 the manpower need will increase roughly by 50%. This increased amount of health workers must help first of all the development of primary health care, the extended and up-to-date application of screening-care-rehabilitation, the manpower needs of special programmes, and the application of wider and new forms of social provision and care. In order to reach it and to decrease the loss caused by mobility, modern and elastic methods for training, regulation and manpower management are needed.

The number of doctors trained will not change essentially. The introduction of the two-graded training for pharmacists seems to be justified and purposeful from a special point of view. The intensive development of health provision needs an increase in the number and proportion of experts with other academic degree than medical (e.g. biophysical, chemical, economic, mathematical).

Increasing the quantitative capacity of training in medical college is not necessary, but a flexible change in the structure of specialities, based on the health needs, is essential (e.g. nurse training on college level, social nurse training). In the field of training the nurses the quantitative and qualitative importance of special secondary school training must be improved together with the improvement of the social situation and working conditions of young nurses.

Permanent post-graduate training concerning all kinds of health manpower is very important. The continuing training of health managers has to be based on the special needs of health provision.

The Role of Government in Health Manpower Planning in Canada

R.B. Holmes, M.D.

Introduction

In discussing the role of government in a country where there is government funding of health care in an open-ended system with few controls on demand, utilization or price, possibly the greatest value in hearing about the Canadian scene is the relation and interplay between the provinces and the federal government in these matters. In this sense there may be some similarities with the relationship of individual countries in Western Europe to each other and to the European Community in respect to manpower problems.

To put health manpower planning in Canada in its proper context we must deal briefly with some factors that apply to the Canadian scene. Having described this context we can then look at manpower planning as it actually occurs in Canada, and as it might occur.

The context factors are six in number:

- geographic and demographic;
- Canada's political constitution;
- the evolution of health care legislation by government;
- the methods of practice of various health care workers;
- the education, qualification and licensing of the medical profession, and relevant for the 1980's,
- government's targets for cost containment.

Geography and Demography

Regarding the first of these, Canada's geography and demography, the country has a population of 24 million which is very unevenly distributed. About 22 million of these live in a long, thin band extending 3,000 miles from east to west, within about 100 miles of the United States border. There are 24 urban centres of over 100,000 population each.

The aggregate population of these centres is almost 15 million people or 60% of Canada's population. Another important factor which is helpful, in examining our neighbour the United States, is that Canada's population is about 1/10 that of the United States.

The country is comprised op 10 provinces and 2 territories. Once again each province has a very uneven distribution of people and natural resources. It ranges from Prince Edward Island the smallest province with a population of 125,000, to Ontario, the industrial heartland of the country with a population of 8½ million.

Some provinces have little manufacturing and few natural resources and others are wealthy in one or both resources. This results in the description of some as have-provinces and others as have-nots. Informally provinces in different regions group together for certain planning and consultation purposes. These fall into five or sometimes four groups, namely the Atlantic provinces, Quebec, Ontario, the Prairie provinces and British Columbia, or more frequently the four western provinces. A practical problem in a country like this is that with the low population density and the large distances, extending over 4½ time zones, face-to-face meetings on the national scene are fewer, and decision making is slower.

Constitution

Regarding its constitution the country was formed 115 years ago by the union of 4 separate British colonies to create Canada. The constitution makes it a confederation with central federal responsibilities such as international affairs, defence, the post office, native people, and national transportation (railways) for example. There is a federal department of health whose function is primarily related to international health, the health of native peoples and health research.

The constitution assigns to the provinces responsibilities which are mainly in the social and cultural areas, and certain local services. Provincial responsibilities therefore include health, education, social services, housing, municipalities and roads.

Apart from its responsibilities, the federal government is playing a major *role* in health and education through the transfer of funds to the provinces to assist them in fulfilling their responsibilities in these areas. The federal government provides about half the cost for health services and post-secondary education. It finances the health research through the Medical Research Council of Canada to the extent of $100,000,000 a year.

Regionalization takes places in some provinces for purposes of health planning.

Health Legislation

Regarding the evolution of health legislation, in 1958 the federal government enacted the Hospital Insurance and Diagnostic Services Act whereby it provided half the funds to cover the cost of operating hospitals, including those medical services which were related to diagnosis within hospitals, laboratory and radiology services.

In 1962 the province of Saskatchewan on its own, introduced an insurance plan to cover medical care services. Its introduction was attended by considerable opposition on the part of the medical profession leading to a 'doctor's strike' of services for 23 days. The outcome to this conflict was that government got its way in general with the exception that doctors were free to opt out of the insurance plan and deal with the patient directly, the patient receiving reimbursement from the government for the bill rendered to the patient by the physician.

In 1964 the federal government created a Royal Commission of Inquiry into health services in Canada. The Royal Commission eventually recommended a national comprehensive plan for personal health services. Two years later the federal government acted on these recommendations and brought into being the Federal Medical Care Act. This legislation made funds available on a 50/50 basis to all provinces which set up and operated *medical care programs* with four basic features.

1. The *scope* of benefits should be, broadly speaking, all the services provided by physicians.
2. The *plan* should be universal. It should cover all residents of a province on uniform terms and conditions.
3. *The administration* of the plan must be public, if the federal government is to contribute, i.e. all private health insurance plans must go out of business.
4. *Transferability of benefits* – when a person moves to another province or is absent from his own province.

In 1977 the federal government enacted the Established Programs Fiscal Arrangements Act, which moved from the previous arrangement of matching funds from the federal government to meet provincial costs on a 50/50 basis, whatever those costs may have been, to a new arrangement of block grants.

In 1979 there was a formal federally initiated *Health Services Review*, which recommended two additional goals:

5. Reasonable compensation for the provider.
6. Uniform terms and conditions of eligibility and coverage.

The Review, in commenting on medical manpower, indicated a ratio of 1 active civilian physician to 666 population.

The report stated 'if present recruitment into the profession continues, that ratio may well be 1 : 300 by the year 2000'. The provincial ministers of

health seeing that figure and relating it to costs, became quite alarmed.
This stimulated further interest by provincial governments into all aspects of medical manpower.

Methods of Practice

Issues concerning medical manpower in Canada are influenced by the type and nature of medical practice. Physicians generally engage in private office practice combined with hospital practice. Most physicians operate on a fee-for-service principle with some hospital-based physicians being paid a salary. Fee schedules for the entire profession are generally developed by each provincial medical association. When the government medical care program came into being it paid a schedule of benefits. This in Ontario for example was originally linked to the fee schedule of the provincial medical association. The benefits initially were 90% of the stated fee schedule, the same percentage that the earlier private doctor-sponsored plan allowed the physician. Physicians were free however to bill the plan and accept the benefit payment as full payment, or they were free to charge the patient an additional amount.

These points illustrate the many freedoms for the practitioners in the system. A practitioner is free to practice where and how he chooses. He is free to choose his method of payment, fee-for-service, capitation or salary. He is free to treat his patient without any concern for the set his own cost of treatment (cost to the patient or to the paying agency, government). He is free to depart from the government established schedule of benefits.

As stated above the schedule began at 90% of the printed fee schedule of the Provincial Medical Association. The setting of the schedule soon evolved into an annual negotiation between the government and the medical association. For example the Ontario Medical Association annually negotiates a percentage increase in government funding for private practice costs. The Association then distributes the increase to the various specialty groups and this is reflected in the individual items in the fee schedule. More recently the Association's dissatisfaction with annual increase is reflected in the fact that the government's schedule of benefits is now only about 73% of the Association's independently set tariff.

Regarding dentistry it is essentially private fee-for- service practice without any government insurance plan. There are many private insurance plans and there is some government support for dental care especially for children. In Canada about 1/3 of the people see the dentist on a regular basis, 1/3 see him only on emergency and 1/3 never see a dentist. Dentists perceive an over-supply of numbers and some are getting into financial difficulty.

Regarding nurses they are traditionally salaried employees usually of a hospital or an employee of a private practising doctor. There are a few nurse practitioner educational programs. The number of nurse-practitioners in the system is minimal in size and impact, the major problem being where and how to employ them. A decade ago there was a perceived oversupply of nurses, which was reflected in a reduction in educational programs. There is now perceived an acute shortage of nurses.

Education

A few comments regarding medical education are relevant for a discussion of medical manpower issues. There are 16 medical schools in Canada. They all undergo a periodic accreditation process which is identical to that for the 116 or so schools in the United States. The standards for accreditation are identical. Each country has its own accrediting body and each has a voting representative on the accrediting body in the other country. The accrediting teams frequently contain a member drawn from the other country. A result is that it is much easier for a Canadian physician to obtain a license to practice in the United States, although easier in some states than in others. This factor is very important when considering medical manpower issues in Canada.

In Canada each province issues a license to practice to anyone from any province or any country who meets the necessary standards via a qualifying examination. A graduate of any school in Canada or elsewhere is eligible to try a pre-licensing examination set by a national body, the Medical Council of Canada. Anyone passing that examination can get a license in any province (except Quebec which has its own licensing examination and organization).

Post-graduate specialty trainees are certified by a national body, the Royal College of Physicians & Surgeons of Canada which covers all specialties except family practice. Trainees in formal university based family practice programs are qualified through the College of Family Practice of Canada. These national certificates of specialty are recognized by each provincial licensing body, the importance of this being that it allows a certificant to charge a specialist fee when practising in a specialty.

Cost-containment

The *political objective* of government is to have a health system with all the ideals of quality, and equality. The realities are that government has an *operational objective*, which is to keep health care costs to their traditional share of the gross national product. Many observers maintain they can only conclude that government's primary concern is cost and that it has only a nominal interest in quality. Using such rough guides as mortality and morbidity, government sees little relationship between quality of care and the numbers of doctors. Government has a perception that there is a direct relationship between the numbers of doctors and the total costs to the system. Dividing the number of doctors into the total cost of the system, some observers have conclude that each additional doctor costs the system $250,000 per year. These factors have lead to another perception by government, that there is a trend to over-supply of physicians.

Health care costs in Canada *have* risen over the past 15 years as a percentage of gross national product. But compared to many other western countries Canada's rate of increase has been well below any of the others. Canada's health care costs have been relatively very well contained. This has gone to the point where over the past 2-3 years increasing pressures are building to allow some easement in cost containment.

In the meantime government continues trying to control costs and to achieve this they have a number of targets for cost-containment. It is important to note that by aiming directly at any one target, government also strikes other targets.

In controlling expenditures the targets are in the hospital sector, the health professional sector, and the educational program sector. The method of containing costs in these sectors is by increasing funding at a rate less than that of inflation.

In Ontario utilization of health services per capita is increasing at a rate of about 2% per year compounded. This is therefore an additional target.

Another approach is in limiting costs through limiting the supply of health manpower hospital beds (or even entire hospital), and facilities such as CT scanners. It is attempting to control prices of inputs for example by limiting the funding allowed for various services such as medical care services.

Government is trying to shift priorities by providing preferential funding to ambulatory and daycare facilities, to shifting of emphasis from medical to allied medical health workers, and decreasing the ratio of medical specialists to general practitioners.

A fourth element in cost is the fact that in three of the ten provinces a significant amount of funding for the system does not come from general tax revenues but from premiums charged to insured individuals (even though in many cases much of the premium is provided as an employer contribution). The theory behind the premiums is that first it relieves those governments of some of the total burden for the health care costs, and secondly that it gives the consumer some awareness that there is a cost element to the provision of health care services.

Health Manpower Planning

Having dealt with a number of context factors within which health manpower planning must operate, one can ask the question: Why do health manpower planning in the first place?. In general terms one does it on the one hand to ensure there is enough health manpower to provide adequate services, and on the other, to avoid having too many health providers from the perspectives of costs and ethics.

If numbers are grossly out of line with needs, broadly defined, the citizens may suffer due to insufficiency. If there are too many, costs may rise far beyond the benefits provided, or the public may be ill-served by competition for patients by too many providers, with unnecessary services being provided.

Approaching manpower planning in this way means that numbers are the prime target, and if looked at from this perspective it is very limited in its value to the system.

One might argue that the prime target should not be manpower planning per se, but policy planning for the provision of the right amount of health service, of the right type provided by the most appropriate health professionals. If so this is the main end to be sought, manpower planning is a secondary target. It is simply the means to an end. What's really happening is that the prime target is being ignored as government tries to manage by crisis rather than manage by policy.

Role of the Federal Government

Regarding the actual role of the federal government in health manpower planning, it seems to be a relatively low priority matter for the federal government.

The one major policy achievement in recent years was the control of immigration of physicians into Canada. This was achieved primarily because of agreement by all the provinces that unlimited immigration of physicians should be controlled. The present policy is that immigration of a physician is allowed usually to fill an academic post of for someone committed to working in an underserviced area. There are still problems because an immigrant family may enter the country and only after arrival does a member identify himself or herself as a physician.

The federal government's role in planning has to do with three national committees, two of which have been operating for about 10 years. The first is the Federal/Provincial Advisory Committee on Health Manpower. It is composed of civil servants and has no decision making powers. It exchanges information but rarely makes specific recommendations, although it did make the recommendation about curtailment of immigration.

The second is the National Physician Manpower Committee which is advisory to the federal government and contains no provincial government members. It is composed primarily of representatives of the various national professional organizations plus federal government representatives. Its function has been to look at projections of need for the next decade.

Neither of these committees is as effective as might be desired. The main benefit is that each is a forum which brings people together to generate and exchange information. They have found it hard to come to grips with the issues since they involved more than one province. It has been felt the committees have been of doubtful value and the federal government is uncertain about what value the provinces get from them.

There is a third ad hoc committee which is chaired by a federal assistant deputy minister. This resulted form the Health Services Review in 1979, already referred to. The specific task is to look at the issue identified in the Review that the country may well be looking at a doctor population ratio of 1 : 300 by the year 2000. The motivation behind creation of the committee was for it to come up with something which would lead to action. So far it has identified some alternative options such as reduction in the numbers of undergraduate students across the country. At the federal level there is a sense that people are not sure where to go next in respect to manpower issues. They feel they do not have a good data base for drawing any conclusions.

Since the federal government is currently paying approximately half the cost of the health system, it continues to have a major and national interest in the health plans. The federal government is particularly concerned about possible erosion of equitable access to health services.

A possible scenario affecting medical manpower is as follows: government is continuing to hold down health expenditures as a percentage of gross national product. Physicians incomes have fallen behind inflation.

Physicians are billing patients above the government benefit level. The federal government claims this will destroy the principle of universal accessability, and has threatened to make funds available to provinces only if they 'outlaw' extra billing. This will lead to confrontations with the medical profession. It may stimulate some to emigrate to the U.S. and others into early retirement. This underscores the impact on health manpower, of policies which may be directed primarily elsewhere in the system.

The most desirable role for the federal government is to enhance its effectiveness in bringing the provinces together and in gathering information. The most desirable role for the federal government is to maintain a national role in support of the health care system, having created that system some fifteen years ago.

Role of the Provincial Government

Regarding the provincial role in health manpower planning, in 1975 the government of Ontario began to relate the number of doctors to the overall costs of the system and concluded that each additional doctor created an additional cost of $250,000 per year. The government of the day accepted the physician supply at the time as being appropriate, and indicated it wished to hold the supply at that level allowing additional physicians only as population increased. It also wished to maintain the existing percentage of specialists in the system. To achieve this it fixed the total number of undergraduate medical students at the 1975 figure, and from time to time it has reduced marginally the number of post-graduate physicians which it would fund through hospital budgets. It created an advisory committee on medical manpower, whose role was primarily that of watchdog and sounding board rather than policy development. More recently one province has reduced the number of post-graduate training positions from 203 to 185. It plans further reductions to 165 and then to 150. In at least 2 provinces government dictates to the universities the numbers of trainees allowed in each specialty training program. In another province the number of trainees was reduced from 2,400 to approximately 2,220. That province is now proposing to eliminate selected entire specialty training programs at one university or another. The province of Ontario has implemented a reduction in post-graduate training numbers of 2% effective July 1982 and proposes further reductions of 5,5% and 5% over the next three years, amount in all to some 450 positions. In one province the minister of Education wishes to increase the size of the undergraduate class whereas the ministry of Health wishes to leave it alone. In another province there has been a 10% reduction in undergraduate numbers, not so much by government decree but by the medical school itself due to constriction on funds. One can only conclude that most of these ad hoc actions by government will not achieve the objectives stated.

What few medical manpower studies have been done are of dubious quality because they have failed to realize the free mobility of physicians from one province to the other, because of a lack of data about supply, or a sense of how to identify true demand. Most of the participants in the planning process are experts in other than the field on manpower planning, or they have special interests at stake. Bloom and Peterson of the University of Pennsylvania have done an extensive review of all medical manpower planning efforts in the United States since the days of Flexner and have pointed out the flaws in methodology and identified the reasons for them.

The most likely possibility is that government will continue to increase its level of control of health manpower in respect to overall numbers, types, distribution and the roles they play. Factors contributing to this control will be methods and amounts of remuneration, and control of the educational programs.

Regarding numbers, the most direct way of controlling them is through the number of licenses that are allowed to be issued in any one year. A lesser level of control would be to limit the number of practitioners who are able to bill the government plan, allowing others to practice but not to bill the plan. Another means of control would be to limit the number who are allowed appointments in a given hospital. Other approaches to control might be changes in legislation to allow other health care workers such as nurses, to perform medical acts and not under medical supervision.

Changes in the amount or method of remuneration of doctors can have a negative effect on manpower numbers by encouraging practitioners to leave a province or the country, and discouraging immigration of others.

At present there seems no way of implementing a manpower policy since no one knows exactly what it should be. One wonders whether the policy should be directed toward medical manpower, or whether to identify the objectives of the health care system which required definition, leaving manpower numbers to float freely within such a defined objectives.

The most desirable role for provincial government is for a clear identification of objectives for the health system in four stages:

1. Overall purpose of the system, its 'raison d'être'.
2. Operational objectives.
3. Then, setting of manpower objectives.
4. Then, planning the strategies for these objectives.

It is essential that if such an approach is to be adopted, that there be national coordination of the various provincial approaches.

At present the province of Ontario does not have such a desirable approach but it does have the mechanism through which such an approach could be realized. I refer to the Ontario Council of Health.

Ontario

The Ontario Council of Health is established by statute as a senior body to advise the minister of Health on health matters and needs of the people of Ontario. It is an independent and impartial body composed of some twenty private citizens. They are appointed to Council based on their ability, experience and interest in the health field. They do not represent any particular professional organization or pressure group. They are appointed by the minister to provide him with policy advice on broad areas of health, and emphasizing the long-term view. The Council operates through special task forces designed with a view to addressing a specific problem. The Council does have a small in-house research capability, and has the ability to contract out research projects of greater scope, which may be needed for the conduct of any given study.

The Council thus has a unique position in the health system. While professional and other specialty organizations and institutions as well as consumers, have the opportunity to advise the minister of Health, it is only the Ontario Council of Health which is in a position to act in an objective way, basing its recommendations on scientifically conducted studies, taking into account the views and judgements of the various groups and formulating a policy proposal which in its judgement is in the best overall public interest. The Council of Health is in fact involved in a major study to advise the minister on medical manpower matters in Ontario, keeping the long-term view in mind.

Its study has two components, first to advise on the government's present intention to reduce post-graduate training positions in Ontario and secondly to advise on any other matter relating to medical manpower. It is attempting to do this keeping in mind government's existing policy to maintain quality but contain costs, to shift emphasis in health care from in-hospital specialty care to ambulatory family practice care, and to make optimal use of nursing and other allied health manpower.

The Council has created a task force of ten individuals including an educationalist, an economist, a health administrator, a former university president, the director of a training program for allied health professionals, a former medical school dean, one nurse and three practising physicians. The task force began by consulting experts in manpower methodology including forecasting. It consulted the special interest groups and it consulted government regarding its objectives. The task force report will go to the parent Council which will send the report out to independent peer review. The Council members will then examine the report and recommend to the minister. Shortly after this it will make public its report to the minister.

One cannot predict the final outcome of the Council of Health's Task Force on Medical Manpower nor the government's response to it. All that can be said at this time is that it is trying to avoid the pitfalls of previous manpower studies, and to examine the problems in the context of the overall objectives of the health care system.

Problems Facing Europe

P.A. Farrelly, M.D.

There have probably always been, and certainly so in modern times, problems of medical manpower. It has always been difficult to match the demand with the supply. This is true, not only of total numbers, but of the specialized areas of practice as well and with the increasing trend towards narrower specialization this has become more acute - one can have poverty of numbers in the midst of plenty.

Likewise there are problems of a distribution nature on a geographic basis within countries and within specialties. In most cases the shortfall is in the more peripheral areas of countries, the pull of the city's bright lights, better and more expensive facilities for practice, better educational and social amenities for families, and generally enhanced earning power often proving irresistable. This leaves many underdeveloped areas short of doctors, especially specialists, despite the allure of good hunting, shooting and fishing country.

There are also manpower problems of an international nature. Some countries appear to be *constantly* over-doctored. Nowadays in Western Europe at least, few are under-doctored.

Where do we start in an attempt to grasp the fundamentals of this complicated and multi-facetted conundrum. It has to do with entry to medical school, with facilities for training, both at undergraduate and post-graduate level, with social security systems and patterns of practice and with earning potential.

Firstly, we can say there is no shortage of candidates for medical school, and unless there is numerus clausus there will be over-supply.

Secondly, we can say that facilities for training in medical school are finite and are usually stretched beyond what is prudent. This can and does lead to excessive numbers of poorly trained doctors.

Thirdly, the facilities for post-qualification training are likewise finite and also are often over-stretched, with the same result.

Fourthly, the system of practice where the family doctor provides primary health care and refers complicated cases to hospital to be treated by consultants appears to lead to a lesser doctor - population ratio as in Ireland and Britain, compared with Belgium and Germany.

Fifthly, the system of practice where a capitation-fee or salary is the norm, as in Britain, seems to need less doctors than where a fee-for-service scheme exists. We can leave the quality of the respective services for further discussion.

The spectre of medical unemployment has been stalking the countries of Europe for the last ten years, and has grown appreciably larger in the last five years. These were set out in a paper prepared by PWG in 1979. In Denmark 13.3.80 327 doctors were out of work and new posts are not being created because of the recession. So they tend to cling on to the present post thus causing a bottleneck. Even in Switzerland, where such a thing was unheard of since the thirties, 30-40 juniors were out of work this year.

So since saturation point has been reached in several countries (anything less than 1 in 500 ratio generally is regarded as saturation and 4 countries are at this point) the only possibility to control the problem and avoid the waste of money and brain power involved in medical unemployment is to limit the numbers going into the system. To give due credit to the profession, they were quite farseeing and several countries took prompt action to cheek the rising graph curve of medical student admission. This rise has now been arrested in all but three EEC member states, but constant attention is necessary to keep the situation under control.

Further, there is some evidence accumulating that medicine as a profession is becoming somewhat less sought, due to the arduous and lengthy training programmes which tend to defer full seniority and earning power to the middle- thirty age, and also due to the unpropitious job prospects of these times.

I congratulate the organizers of this conference for their initiative. They have provided a useful forum for the discussion of this topic of such vital importance to our profession and have assembled a variety of speakers well qualified to make positive contributions to its solution. This must lie, for the future, very largely in the field of stricter application of numerus clausus in those countries which have it, and in making every effort to encourage and persuade those who so far have not introduced it to do so.

Furthermore, efforts should be made in each country and perhaps also at the level of the EEC to improve the distribution pattern of doctors, largely by providing health facilities for the practice of medicine in the more remote areas, and perhaps financial incentives as well. In addition efforts should be made to increase the attractiveness of less popular specialties which will redound to the advantage of both the doctors and the population they serve.

General Discussion

Aarimaä: asked dr Forgács whether he had calculated the contribution of the 60%-70% female doctors to the medical care and compared this with the contribution of their male colleagues.

Forgács: estimates that the total (life-long) productivity of a female doctor is lower than that of a male doctor, because they have different life styles. In Hungary, in the average population, the retirement age for women is 54, for men it's 60.
Leer: suggested, dividing possibilities and desirabilities, to deal firstly with the problem of manpower in view of education and quality of health care and secondly to analyse the problem of the tremendous costs of health care. Having determined the desired functions of health care, thirdly the question arises 'how much can we afford and how much are we willing to pay to our doctors'. Science suffers when economy plays too big a role too soon in this discussion.
Holmes: agreed that dr Leer has put forward fundamental points. Manpower planning appears to be a mere manipulation of numbers. Of course, it's important, keeping in mind the economic realities, to identify the kind of system, with the suitable kind of health care providers, that society really needs. Following this, an appropiate number of physicians should be fixed, but this may be very difficult to do. In short, dr Holmes confessed that he himself couldn't provide the answers to these important questions.
Farrelly: also agreed with the former speakers, although he stressed that economy and science are inseparable. He illustrated this statement with an example.
Wells: emphasized that the concepts of health and health care are mixed during this conference. He stated that, certainly the number of doctors per head of the population is important in respect to the quality of health care. He wondered whether the medical profession should not try and persuade governments to spend more money on health care. Eventually he asked dr Holmes about methods of controlling immigration of doctors in Canada.
Holmes: explained that immigration of doctors in Canada is limited by use of a kind of 'point-system', set up by the federal government and based on economical and functional criteria. Of course the system is not perfect. Furthermore he agreed with dr Wells on the need to spend more money on health care by the various governments, especially in Canada and the United Kingdom.

McNally: asked the members of the panel about their opinions on the impact on employment of an open market system, such as in Canada, and a closed specific nominated post system like in Ireland and the UK. Secondly he asked dr Farrelly as the chairman of the ACMT about his opinion on the qualitative consequences on education and health care of the Danish shift-system, whereby a specific limited number of hours is worked to give employment to the excess number of junior doctors.
Farrelly: said that of course in a fixed post system unemployment will hit quicker than in an open market system, as here doctors will probably almost automatically share the amount of work. Answering dr McNally's

second question dr Farrelly stated that the ACMT emphasized that, to ensure the quality of training, junior doctors should however have the opportunity to get the necessary experience to become a competent doctor.

Holmes: commented on Farrelly's statement by saying that, since the Canadian government tried to hold doctors incomes down by reducing the fees, the doctors started seeing more patients in order to maintain their incomes. In doing so the doctors create their own employment.

SESSION V:

WORKSHOPS

Introduction

Health manpower planning should be an integral part of health planning and can be defined as the determination of the production, deployment and use of (medical) manpower in the right numbers and qualifications at the right place and time, with the requisite skills and motivation to deliver optimal health care to the population. Health manpower planning is more than making quantitative estimates of manpower needs and supply, and the balance between these two subjects. Ideally, the health manpower planning process should consist of:

- a description of a conceptual framework;
- an analysis of the relationship of manpower planning to the national health planning;
- an improvement of the knowledge of factors influencing the quality and effectiveness of manpower planning.

This ideal situation has not yet been achieved. The main goal of the workshops is the awakening of the necessity for the planning process.

Health manpower planning is a purposeful activity, which plays a major role in the interrelationship between the health care system and the health manpower training system (figure 1).

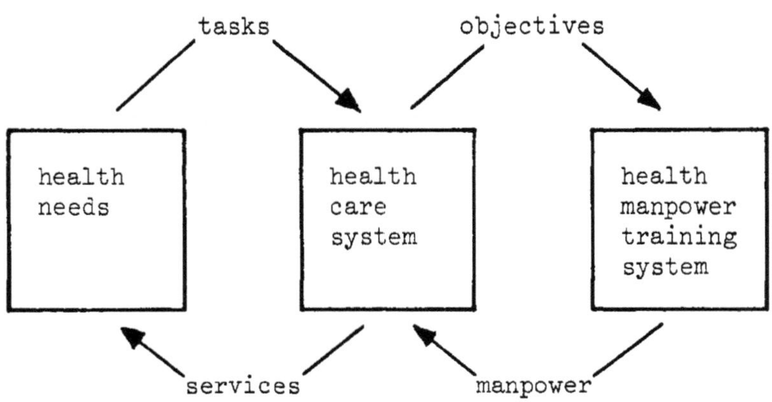

Figure 1 The Process of Health Manpower Planning

Health manpower planning is a directed activity with strategic purposes, and has to be based upon a situative report on existing manpower and services. Many factors are influencing the future supply and requirements of manpower (figure 2). This outline represents the theoretical basis for the distribution of topics and themes for the workshops during the conference.

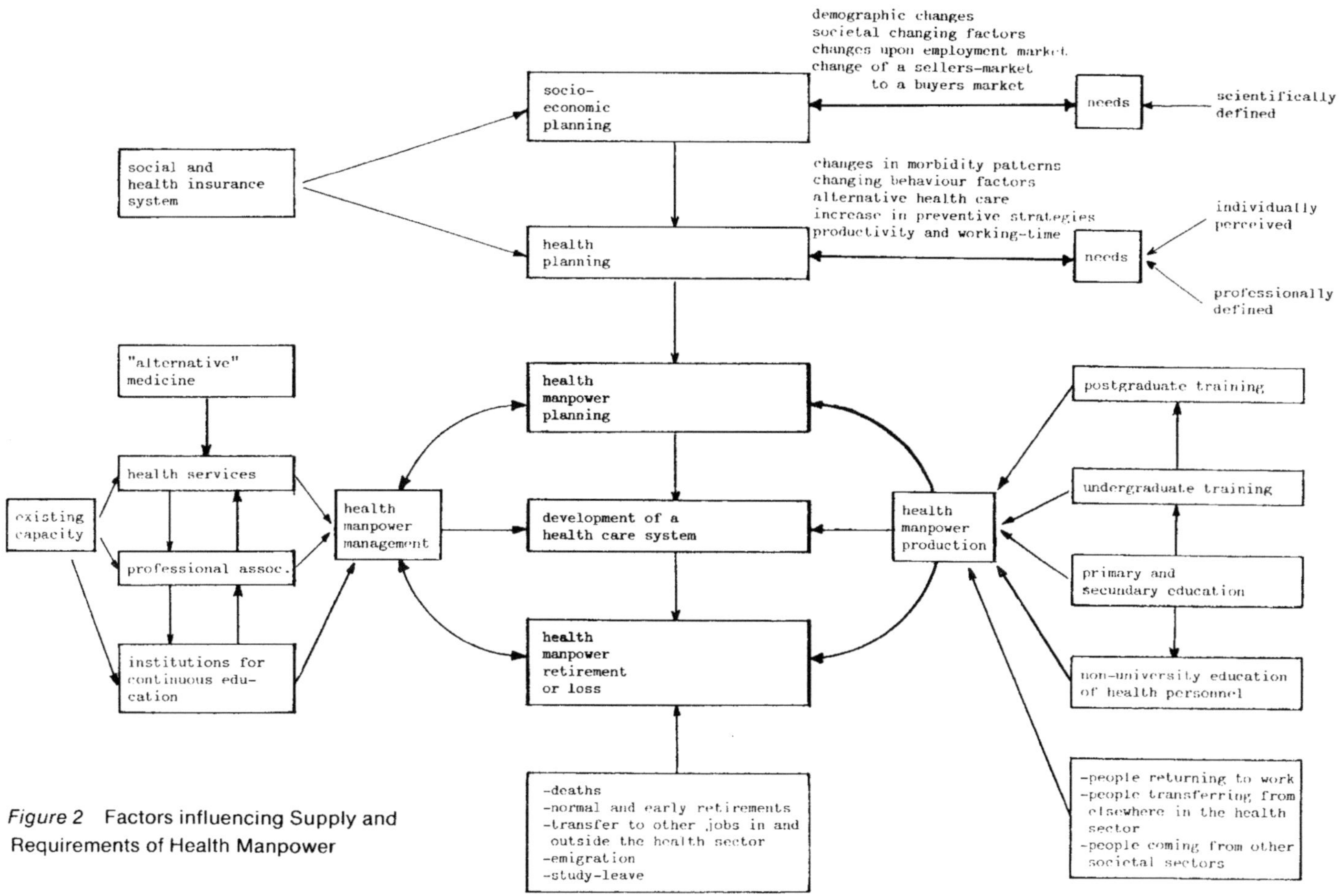

Figure 2 Factors influencing Supply and Requirements of Health Manpower

Task and design of the workshops

The workshops intend to allow the participants to formulate practical advices regarding the process of health manpower planning. Therefore workshop participants will discuss elements of the health manpower planning system. Based upon the results of the workshop discussions, conclusions and recommendations will be formulated during the final session of the conference. The strength and the applicability of the final conclusions and recommendations will follow from the contributions to and the degree of consensus of the participants in the discussion. These conclusions and recommendations will be submitted to the national and European authorities.

Each workshop will deal with one (major) aspect of the whole problem; together they will give an integrated view of the health manpower planning process. The products of the workshops relate to:

- the definition of the needs;
- the development of the health care system;
- the development of the educational system;
- the interrelationship between the health care system and the educational system;
- the career planning of the individual as part of the manpower planning process.

Each topic will be discussed in two groups simultaneously. Since each group will report the results of their deliberations, discussion between groups is also possible. The groups will consist of participants from various countries to accentuate the importance of manpower planning at the supranational level.

Workshop I: Definition of the Needs

An important goal of the process of health manpower planning is to relate the need for health care of the society to the need for health workers in that society. Because we are dealing with an existing health care system, ideal needs and demands are not the indicators to determine the need for health manpower. Far more important are shifts and changes in the needs and demands in the different parts of the health care system and between various categories of health workers, for example:

- the shift between general (non-hospital) and hospital practice;
- the shift of tasks and workload between physicians and ancillary personnel, or between members within one professional group (e.g. medical specialists);

- the importance and influence of 'alternative medicine' to patients, doctors and the 'official' health care system;
- the shift in appreciation of different health workers by the clients.

These examples are expressions of a dynamic process of defining the needs of health care. Health needs can be perceived individually or in groups of patients, but they can also be defined professionally and scientifically.

Questions to be discussed

1.1. Which changes in professional activities and in the science of medicine can be identified in relation to changes in needs?
1.2. Which existing or new indicators or data must be obtained, to estimate the correct number of physicians needed?
1.3. What are the indicators that reflect the changing needs? How can they be identified?
1.4. Defining the needs is a continuous dynamic process. Is it possible for the health professions to identify shifts in health needs in time? In which way can the process of defining the needs be organized? Who is responsible for controlling this process?

Report from workshop I
reporters: dr Reerink (NL) and dr Aärimaä (SF)

Much time was spent on the various current definitions of the needs. An important reason for confusion is the use of more than one scientific or pseudo-scientific term, for instance needs described in terms of health and disease, and needs described as interventions or appliances. So describing the needs in other possible ways, for instance in terms of economical costs, is let out of consideration. The problem of the definition of the needs was solved by translating it, or using the word, 'requirements'. In doing so one could define the parameters, which can help to determine the number of required health workers, and, especially, of physicians. It would also be possible to indicate the systems or data by which one can monitor the changes and shifts of these parameters. The requirements of physician manpower are then determined by demographic developments, social developments and developments in medicine and technology.

The demographic developments are given by the parameters birth-rate, death-rate and by the changing pattern of diseases. These parameters determine not only the number of physicians required, but tell us also something about the functions and tasks of these doctors. It is believed, that in future more attention has to be paid to the care of the elderly and disabled and to the improvement of existing treatment-schedules. In Western countries we have perhaps reached the maximum of the screening possibilities and for reasons of prevention no more doctors are required. The influences of the present prevention and surveillance programmes on the (declining) need for hospital beds are however uncertain. Monitoring these demographic parameters is a matter of more epidemiological studies and of health- and health services surveys. Items to be monitored are the numbers of birth, death and diseases (and especially shifts in disease-patterns), working schedules of the different health services, cost-benefit analyses of treatment-patterns, and so on.

The social developments are given by the parameters: structure of the population, influences and tasks of other professions (psychologists, social workers, para-medical personnel, etc.), the situation on the employment-market (rates of employment and unemployment), the tendency of more part-time work in medicine, the male/female ratio of physicians, the duration of the work week and the tendencies to more non-patient related activities, like education, administration and research. These developments influence directly the requirement of health personnel. Macro-sociological factors, such as patients behaviour, care seeking behaviour, the rate of functional diseases and the function of the health service in regard to other social institutions (e.g. the insurance against disablement), are not just indicating new shifts in functions of doctors, but are also indicating that more doctors are needed for other than strictly defined somatic-medical tasks. Sometimes it seems doctors are being used only for social contacts by lonely people.

Monitoring these social parameters is very extensive and complex. Not only a good registration and understanding of the functioning of the employment-market is needed, but also continuous (sociological) research of changing behaviour patterns inside the population and categories of professional labour. For instance what is 'socio-economic stress' to the population? What is the influence of the 'threat' of a real loss of income? It seems that in the present economic situation, these factors are increasing, and are creating a greater demand for medical help. What is the influence of the fear for a nuclear bomb dropping? What is the influence of more leisure-time? Perhaps the registration of some psychiatric diagnoses (and changes in the number of psychiatric diagnoses) is a parameter for monitoring social developments, which influence the requirements of (special categories of) doctors.

Developments in the medical sciences and technology can have implications to the requirement of other kinds of doctors. Although one cannot forecast these developments, it is possible that more medical specialities will develop and more specialists of a particular kind are needed. The same situation can be encountered in the pharmaceutical industry, and more (and more qualified) doctors are needed for health administration and management. No clear monitoring system for these parameters exists. Perhaps this should be developed.

In summary it is concluded that the demographic developments alone will not lead to an increasing demand of doctors. Especially social developments with the changes in behaviour patterns of the population changes in medical practice, and, to a lesser extent, developments in medicine and technology, will increase the demand of for physicians in future.

Who whould be responsible for controlling this process? The demographic developments should be monitored and guided by the health-authorities, the social developments by cooperation between the health- and employment-authorities and the medical associations. The developments in medicine and technology should be monitored by the medical scientific societies, who would have to report on a regular basis to the authorities and professional associations. New legislation and a formal organization of this process is therefore likely to be needed.

Workshop II: Development of the Health Care System

In most European countries two major developments are going on inside the health care system:

- expansion of the care, with an increasing differentiation;
- division of the care system in primary health care and hospital care.

The expansion of the care system has taken place in a period of growing economic possibilities. But in the present economic situation the sellers-market changes into a buyers-market. Now the need to direct the development of the health care system is becoming more apparent. Can in this situation the mechanism of the free market control the development of the care system?

In primary health care in industrialized countries, psychological and social aspects of health care are becoming more important in general. In the hospital care a still increasing number of specialities can be seen. Cooperation and interrelationships between primary health care and hospital care have become increasingly difficult in recent years.

Questions to be discussed:

2.1. Which developments in primary health care and in hospital care should be related to the manpower production system?

2.2. Which developments, if any, related to the inter relationships between primary health care and hospital care and their consequences to health manpower planning, can be expected in the near future?

2.3. Which market factors, related to health care, play a role in the shift from an expanding economy to a limited economy, in regard to health manpower planning?

2.4. What problems can be expected when a 'free enterprise' health care system is changed into a government controlled system?

Report from workshop II
reporters: dr Kielty (UK) and dr Gentleman (UK)

The participants of this workshop felt, that they should begin by restating the questions asked in the introductory paper:

1. What is at present the relationship between the nature of doctors' jobs and the planning of the number and distribution of doctors?
2. How will this relationship develop and will it be changed in the years ahead?
3. What factors limit or control the development of health care systems?
4. How can a system based on free enterprise be transformed into one where there is central planning of medical manpower?

The participants felt that it was important to state at the onset their belief, that the total level of health care provision is a political decision, largely determined by economic considerations. This is especially so with primary care. However, the distribution of doctors is something on which the medical profession can exercise a degree of control.

The workshop distinguished clearly between long-term planning aims and short-term crisis management. The latter must vary according to the nature and scale of the problem in each country, and the machinery and resources available to meet the problem. Medical manpower planning is a long-term objective, and this means that we are living with decisions that were taken ten, fifteen, even twenty years ago. It requires little insight to appreciate that these decisions were not free of faults; indeed, we are gathered here to confront the problems that have grown from them. The lesson we must draw is that the outcome of plans must be monitored continuously, to allow adjustments to be made for changing economic or other circumstances. This presupposes that the planning machinery is geared to monitoring developments and that the plan itself is flexible enough to allow for adjustments. In some countries such machinery already functions well; in others, as was found in this workshop, the machinery is non-existent or ineffective, and the result is an uncontrolled proliferation of doctors and an inefficient use of material and human resources.

How do we achieve control? It was felt that a rational approach to the problem would require an analysis of what doctors actually do. This can only be done within individual countries, because of the different organizational structures of the health services. For example, such an analysis varies with the division into primary care and hospital care, between the private and public sectors, between the medical and paramedical and administrative professions, and between the career grades and doctors in training. There are many complicating factors, such as the changing working hours of all doctors, the role of women and overseas doctors, and the demands of new technology. In some countries, the traditional role of the doctor as the healer is being slowly replaced by a role of manager and leader of a team, with increasingly complex administrative duties. These factors are not static, but vary over time, and no generalizations can ever be made in manpower planning.

Of the developments affecting manpower production the over all level of provision that any country wishes to make concerning health care, is of primary importance. This is a political decision that needs to be made by the social institutions rather than by it's doctors, particularly when primary care should be available to all citizens.

Other developments that have implications on manpower production are:

- new arrangements for referral: referral to hospital care by the patients themselves or by general practitioners only (apart from emergencies);
- implications on the training programmes for trainees and trainers manpower. There exists a need for additional manpower to take account of the needs for flexibility as programmes develop (to allow for change of course);
- the type of work undertaken by doctors after basic training;
- in particular the developments in primary care have implications on the training programmes and also on the required manpower.

It was felt that a reversal of the current trend towards hospital-based medicine would be cost-effective and permit the redistribution of scarce resources. This would be particularly applicable in certain patient groups, such as the aged and the handicapped, who would be better looked after in the community than in hospital, and at a lower cost to the nation. The division of health care itself into primary and secondary branches is artificial, and it was felt that there should be better coordination between these two sectors, and more overlap of the function of doctors. A problem here is the different structure of primary and hospital health services in different countries, making comparisons difficult.

Three new developments related to the interrelationship between primary health care and hospital care were seen. The first one being the development of comprehensive primary care. The second one was the extent to which primary care will become integrated with secondary care in hospitals. For instance to which extent general practitioners are going to work in hospitals. This tendency could be stimulated by the more comprehensive training of general practitioners. On the other hand, special categories of patients, like the mentally handicapped and the aged, would profit more by primary care than by hospital care. This may mean a shift from secondary to primary health care. A third development in the interrelationship between the two categories of health care is the tendency to shorten the patients stay in hospital. But as far as shifts from the hospital care back into the primary care are concerned, this workshop saw some essential restrictive conditions. There is a need for adequate primary care standards, for these could be over-leveled. Also there is a need for adequate paramedical and community support. More nursing services and possibly social services. Will the patients, however, accept these new concepts of care? Patients acceptability is a problem in some countries. Patients acceptability and expectancies limit the possibilities of development in primary care. Therefore there is a (new?) considerable role for health education.

The influence of patient demand varies considerably, and is hard to quantify; we have already heard about the pitfalls of using demand as a measure of need. The impact of an exploding technology has marked effects on the nature of many doctors' jobs, and also affects patient demands, by making the hitherto impossible quite feasible. Here again, however, the realities of economic constraints overshadow all other factors.

The maintenance of levels of expenditure on health care, which were adequate in real terms, depends on a political decision. The governments may have to reset their priorities and – in some countries – to increase the percentage of the gross national product which they spend on health. Of course this will be difficult, particularly with economic restraints, growing unemployment and the demand for lower taxe. Growth in health care should not be singled out for restriction, because we are entering a near limited economy, but the amounts of money spent on health care should be reduced, pro rato, with everything else.

The consensus in this workshop was that private medicine is less cost-effective than a national health service; in addition, a system of health insurance lends itself less well to overall planning than one based on a national health service. Economic constraints are hindering the natural progression of doctors in training in many countries, and are contributing to the difficulties of making plans for tomorrow on the assumptions of today.

Other problems, which can be expected when a 'free enterprise' health care system is changed into a national health service, are the maintenance of standards, the redistribution of manpower, the increase of bureaucracy and the resistance of professionals. This resistance springs from the doctors' traditional idea of free enterprising a practice. Interferences of government in free consultation, making diagnoses, treatment and prescription of drugs, is hardly accepted. Great difficulties will arise concerning the redistribution of manpower and services to increase the resource accessibility. Furthermore problems may arise form the funding (tax levels before and after the change of the health care system). The population may have to provide a larger part of their income (tax) to meet the costs of a new system.

Resistance to change from within the medical profession is a stumbling block to progress. The coefficient of inertia of doctors should never be underestimated. As well as an instinctive antipathy to change, such resistance may stem from self-interest or from genuine doubts about the wisdom of proposed changes. The cooperation of the profession, if not essential, is certainly most desirable in the establishment and use of machinery to plan medical manpower in response to changing needs and changing circumstances. It should be realized by all concerned that the profession regards itself as the guarantor of standards in health care, and indeed may be the only body qualified to act in this way.

Workshop III: Development of the Educational System

The educational system, especially that part that produces physicians, forms an essential component of the health manpower system. An important characteristic of the training system is its duration, e.g. for medical specialists twelve to fourteen years. A permanent tension can exist between the planning and the actual production of physicians, where for instance the production process is autonomously defined by criteria other than those of the health care system and is fixed for many years. For example the number of medical students admitted to the faculties of medicine will be influenced by today's health care developments. However, after finishing their professional training, they can find themselves in a situation totally different from that when they started their medical education.

The prolonged period of education, the so-called leadtime, with the restricted possibilities to change the educational programmes, is a key-issue in the educational system regarding manpower planning.

Questions to be discussed:

3.1. Which developments can be expected with regard to the organization, structure, duration and content of the health manpower educational system, especially for physicians?

3.2. Is it possible to influence the number of physicians in different categories during the training period of 12-14 years? If so, in which manner and by whom?

3.3. Is it, based upon ethical, social and financial aspects, acceptable to admit students to an educational process of 12-14 years duration and, at the end of the training period, deny them access to the health care system?

Report from workshop III
reporter: dr O'Callaghan (Eire)

There is a need in every country for a competent body to deal with standards in quality of medical education and planning speciality training programmes. These bodies would contain adequate representation of practising doctors and doctors who teach the trainees. There should also be coordination of these bodies between member states.

These advisory bodies would recommend and carry out accreditation and inspections of hospital posts, assess the qualifications of the trainees, the academic and practical content of the course undertaken by the trainee. Utilization of non-university hospitals in order to ensure enough clinical experience in the form of paid posts for all specialist trainees is necessary. The training authorities already mentioned would play a major role in ensuring that quality standards apply in both university and non-university hospitals and in planning programmes which would enable trainees to gain experience in both types of hospital.

In order to produce a wide variety of doctors, suitable for all types of medical work - an initial selection into medical school - a candidate should be looked at as an entire person. Their academic ability should not be the only consideration. Cultural, sporting, and social abilities should also be considered. It is suggested at this point that a study to determine the criteria that are used for entry into medical school, might be a worthwhile venture.

Career guidance is a very necessary thing. This should be available to both individuals and to a group as a whole.

It should be part of both school and medical school facilities - giving information as to national needs and trends.

We are all aware that there are 'popular' and 'unpopular' specialities - it is suggested that maybe some of the unpopular specialities could have their academic respectability raised with improved working conditions. Perhaps more exposure to these 'under subscribed' specialities during the medical school curriculum may improve the recruitment - maybe even increasing salaries in the specialities particularly when they are situated in unpopular parts of the country.

The 'Common Trunk' concept of training is also a necessary mechanism. It is both progressive and on going. People during the early stages of specialist training could be made aware of job opportunities in various fields of medicine and hopefully would be translocated into these - by this means a proportion of people would be taken away, from the over-populated 'popular' specialities. As before, exposure to as many different specialities as possible at undergraduate level is desirable - but it is often left too late. There needs to be some flexibility in training programmes to allow changing from one speciality to another. Finally we must ask ourselves: are we becoming overspecialized?

The third question can be answered simply: – it is not acceptable. It can be argued that it is a fundamental right of man to choose the discipline that he wishes to study, however, this right does not necessarily quarantee him a job at the end of his study period. It would seem that a sense of proportion in this issue is necessary as in many systems doctors leave and go elsewhere. There maybe temporary 'bulges' in manpower levels but we should not be too inflexible as at any one time we are planning for ten to fifteen years ahead. However, it does seem illogical to go on admitting to medical school if a saturation point has been reached at post graduate level. Restriction into medical school has in many countries only taken place on a very small scale. In some countries intake has increased. If, however, restriction of numbers entering medical school has been enforced – and although these numbers may still be too large – it was felt that the government was bound to provide the means for one to practise one's profession.

During medical education there should be options for changing from one speciality to another or even changing from medicine to a new field. A system such as this would basically be correcting the malproportion that exists within specialities in general.

Further types of training have been inaugurated in some countries i.e., a basic education in certain allied medical subjects – one course leading to qualification as a doctor (vocational training), the other type of education leading to be a worker within the health care system – other than a doctor. This latter form of training then gives the person the option to pursue a totally different career outside medicine after finishing this basic training course – if they so desire. The person who has graduated as a doctor can then enter vocational training – in order to receive specialization.

Overall having subjected students to 12-14 years of education and leaving them jobless at the end of this time is unacceptable – however the situation is changing from an unregulated system to a regulated one. It is up to us as a community to see that these regulations provide the best for the future of medicine and health care in the European Community as a whole.

Workshop IV: Interrelationship between the Health Care System and the Educational System

Health manpower planning is a directed activity relating the needs, defined by the health care system, to the output of the educational system. The final aim of manpower planning is to bring into balance the need for and the supply of manpower. The interaction between these systems needs coordinated activities at the national, and often supranational, policy-making level.

Questions to be discussed

4.1. How can coordination be organized between the health care and the educational systems in relation to manpower planning?

4.2. Is the government a participant by necessity in this coordination? If so, at what level: local, regional, national, supranational? Under which conditions, and what is the role of these legislative bodies?

4.3. In most industrialized countries the health care system is conducted as a public utility and the health manpower training system as a government controlled system. What can be expected from health manpower planning trapped between these two systems?

Report from workshop IV
reporters: dr Shivananda (NL) and dr Bollag (H)

In order to come to grips with the task of defining the interrelationship between the health care system and the educational system, it was agreed that the question of resource/money should be included in the considerations, and that, instead of answering each subquestion individually one should proceed such as to embrace all three questions under one cover. Organically all the three questions are related.

Inspired by the Scottish model, which was found to be more or less paralleled in other European countries (e.g. The Netherlands), the discussion was led around the following scheme of three interacting bodies (figure 3).

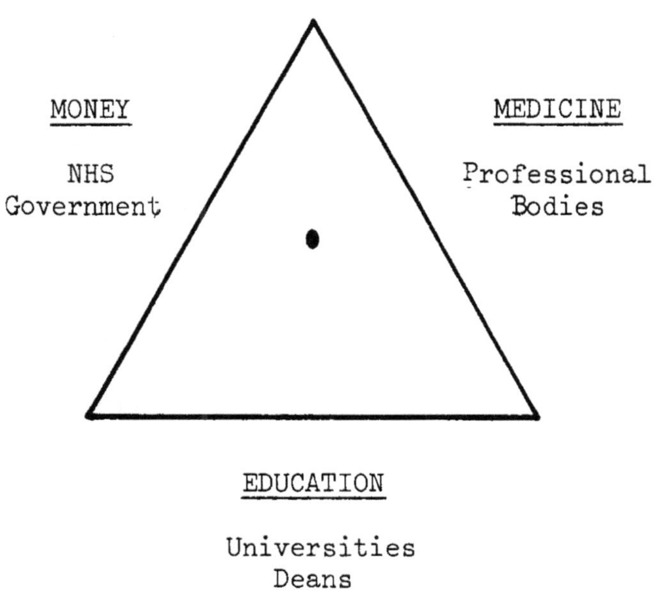

Figure 3 Tripartite Council

The 'Tripartite Council' consists of representatives of three interacting bodies. One is Medicine itself, which is represented by professional bodies; the second is Education, represented by the (deans of) universities; and the third body is the Money providing source, for instance the government or the national health service. The delegates meet in the Council, a kind of sapiential authority, meaning it would discuss by wisdom and value judgement. Each of the representative bodies makes its contributions to policy and acts according to the guidelines the Council agreed upon. The Council's decisions are based on consensus and it doesn't give directives. This would be more acceptable and effective than the present set-up where authoritative statements are made by each of the constituting bodies separately, and where each body is giving its own directives. This kind of set-up of cooperation must be dynamic and flexible. Such a tripartite council would automatically (through exchange of information) deal with some of the following issues (each issue conditioned by the demand and need of the other two bodies): health manpower numbers, most appropriate type of education, aspects of quality of education and adequate funding.

As a proposition of continuous and flexible cooperation between the health care system, the educational system and the financing system, one can answer the last two questions in detail.

The government must inevitably be a participant, because it is the authority which, in varying degrees and depending on the political system, allocates the funds, either at the local, regional or national level.

In view of the extreme difficulties to cope with the most complex matter of interrelationship between the health care system, the educational system and the provision of financies on a national level, it seemed unrealistic to the participants of this workshop to institute a coordinating and directing body at a supranational level, at least at present. In addition it was felt that as each country was heavily pressed by its own difficulties, other problems would be faced in the process of founding a supranational body: language barriers, protectionism and nationalistic feelings, cultural diversities, etc. However, the participants proposed the immediate creation of an information exchange body on the supranational level, the EC-level. The Regional Office for Europe of the World Health Organization may be able to play an important role here.

With regard to the last question: In the set-up of a tripartite council, health manpower planning is not so much trapped between systems, but becomes apart of it.

Workshop V: Relationship between Individual Career Planning and Health Manpower Planning on the 'Macro Level'

The health care professions have to fulfil the needs in the different fields of health care. This functioning must be defined, typified and planned, in terms of both quantity and quality. Ultimately, individual career planning is necessary. Only by planning the future functions can the career risk for the individual student be minimized. On the other hand students should be advized to remain flexible in their career planning and job expectations.

Questions to be discussed

5.1. How can the various functions be described in the health care field, both quantitatively and qualitatively?
5.2. Who decides which functions shall be exercized and at which level?
5.3. Who is responsible for the selection of students for specific training and the selection of the newly qualified specialists? Which selection criteria should be used?
5.4. What is the present state of individual career planning among physicians? How does personal career planning interfere with manpower planning?

Report from workshop V
reporters: dr Naaborg (NL) and dr McNally (UK)

The questions about defining the various functions in health care and the decision which function will be exercized, came together and were really difficult to deal with. The view of the participants of this workshop was, that, in spite of there being many different aspects to health care and many different, although complementary health care professions, historically *doctors* have defined the functions, quantitatively as well as qualitatively. At present this shouldn't be so any more. In the current medical professional training, in particular with its inward looking aspects, this appears to be undesirable. The decisions which functions will be exercized and at what level, should be made by a broader group of representatives from the field of politics, economy, medicine and patients.

The necessity of the team approval at a more particular and clinical level, was discussed. The view was that the physician, although ultimately clinically responsible, should not as a fundamental right be the team-leader, but the leadership should vary, depending on the subject being discussed at the time. Also under this heading – teams versus clinical responsibility – vocational commitments were discussed. Doctors shouldn't have to work an excessive number of hours.

In selection, both for special training and for new specialities, it was agreed that academic standards should take second place to an over all assesment of all the activities of the individual. This selection should be made by an independent panel. With the present selection criteria in the highly industrialized world, the quality of health care is of such a level that the question is not relevant any more. In selecting trainees for medical specialization, also the suggestion was made that the selection panel should include a trainee who is close to the end of his training. This trainee should assist in identifying the suitable candidates.

At present, individual career planning among physicians is unguided, which is undesirable. Students and trainees start usually without guidance. Here the teacher has a double responsibility: first each teacher has a responsibility towards the education of his students and trainees. He has to identify the fields of medicine that have good career prospects for the trainees/doctors-to-be. Secondly he has a global responsibility towards his profession: he has to assess the abilities of his trainees, but also he has to bear in mind the possibilities in numbers in each speciality.

An important matter is that politicians can always criticize the medical profession as a group, as long as there are vacant posts.

CONCLUSIONS AND RECOMMENDATIONS

Conclusions

A.R. Tarlov, M.D.

Before beginning the main body of my summary I would like to thank dr Eric Vrijland and the staff, and particularly mrs De Groot, for the excellent organization of this symposium.

To summarize a conference of this sort can be an amusing exercise. For those of you who are frequenters of the cinema you may recall a Japanese movie called 'Rashomon' in which there were five men all of whom simultaneously observed the same event. In the movie each of the five men told their account of what they had seen. Each of the five tales was remarkably different. Reporting of an experience is a very individualistic affair in which we often take liberty in reporting our individual interpretations. I hope that my summary of this conference does not appear strange or unfamiliar to you. We did participate in the same event but our subjective interpretations may be different. Also consider, of course, that you have for the past half hour been to the 'Limburgian Tea Party', but I haven't. Now that I know what a Limburgian Tea Party is I assume that you are ready to accept almost anything.

In this summary report I have divided my comments into three categories:

A) a statement of the *problem*,
B) a description of those items about which I perceive a *consensus* has been reached, and
C) from the consensus two important *recommendations* can be deduced.

A. The Problem

The problem can be succinctly stated in three short sentences. The rate of production of physicians is not closely related to the need for physician services in most countries. One result has been over-production of physicians, an aggregate surplus of physicians either present or impending, and physician unemployment. Because of the European Economic Community directive of 1976 this problem is transnational and transeuropean.

Those three sentences define the problem. They are in fact paraphrases from the opening remarks of dr Eric Vrijland and they have been echoed by most speakers at the conference.

B. Consensus

There are thirteen points upon which there has been general agreement or consensus. I do not wish to imply unanimity. By consensus I mean a collective opinion, general agreement, or a majority view. I believe that consensus has developed at this conference on many topics. Although individual participants may wish to dissociate themselves from some of these opinions I suggest to you that there has developed general agreement on the following thirteen items.

1. *The Problem* – As stated above.
2. *A surplus of Doctors is Undesirable* – This is remarkable. In the United States there is disagreement on this subject. Many Americans, particularly the economists, believe a surplus would be advantageous.
3. *Causes of the Problem* – General agreement has been expressed that throughout the 1940's, 50's and 60's the health services sector and the education system enjoyed unprecedented growth in terms of the funds made available for their development. The people of your countries have placed a very high value on health services. Governments have assigned a high priority to expanding health services and health education. The current problem owes its origin not to any diminution in the value your people place on health, but rather to the world economic recession and the need to restrain expenditures for health care and health education. This problem has lead to a restriction of growth and in some cases to a diminution in services.
4. *Integrated Planning* – General agreement was reached on the desirability of a comprehensive program which would integrate planning of the health education system with planning for the health services system.
5. *Plan for all Health Provider Personnel* – Wide agreement was expressed on the need to integrate manpower planning for doctors, nurses, and other health services personnel.
6. *Methodology* – Methodologies for estimating supply and requirements for physician services have been developed. There has been a great deal of discussion about defining the term 'needs'. Despite that discussion each country reporting at this conference has substituted in place of needs a proxy value such as a percentage of the gross national product, physician to population ratio or some other measurement of requirements which satisfied the planning function in their respective countries.

I wish to pause to make a comment about the question of needs or the requirements for physicians services. We are on the threshold of an important advance in health manpower planning. A definition of needs which has operational parameters can be derived from the 1977 World Health Organization resolution 'Health for All' in which the objectives of health care revolve around the concept of attaining full economic and social productivity for each individual. Health services researchers are in process of converting the traditional needs concept, based on prevention of morbidity and mortality, to a new concept based on the functional status of the individual in terms of their economic and social productivity and their neuromuscular, intellectual, and emotional functioning in their natural environment. Efficacy of medical intervention will be assessed in terms of restoring function or maintaining optimal function. This development has the potential of leading to a much more useful discussion of 'needs' five years from now than is possible presently.

7. *Fascination* - I have been amused by what appears to be fascination by you and your European colleagues on the subject of women in medicine? Many speakers spoke to this subject from the podium. Many participants conversed informally in the corridors and over lunch with interest, curiosity, pride, worry, bewilderment and in brief, fascination.
8. *The Entry Point* - Agreement was expressed that the best mechanism for control of manpower development is at the point of entry to the medical education system. Many other alternatives were discussed, some of them aimed at short term correction. But regulation of the first year class size emerged as the preferred mechanism for the long term.
9. *Short Term Correction* - There has been agreement expressed relative to the urgent need for short term planning and action, a need which has been accentuated by the rising unemployment rate of physicians in several European countries.
10. *Trans-National Approach* - Your presence at this meeting indicates your understanding that well intentioned national actions may be undermined by actions taken in good faith by other nations of the Community. Long term planning requires transnational cooperation and coordinated action.
11. *Social Consensus* - A very sensitive appreciation has been expressed at this conference that a broad social consensus must be constructed before any significant action can be taken. That point in regard to public opinion or national acceptability was expressed by many individuals. Awareness of the requirement for social consensus makes it imperative that planning not only take place at the transnational and national levels but also within the regions of your countries.
12. *Government Action Needed* - No disagreement was expressed relative to the need for legal, legislated, or centralized approaches to this

problem. That came as a surprise to me because in my country the opinion of physicians, legislators, and government personnel is in the opposite direction looking toward the private sector for most of the corrective action. Nonetheless, at this conference most if not all participants look to the governments for resolution.

13. *Infra-National Participation* – The last point that I will make in regard to consensus is that infra-national or regional organizations must have strong or powerful input into the planning and implementation of policies discussed at this conference.

C. Recommendations

It seems clear that both short term and long term actions must be undertaken.

Short term because physician unemployment requires urgent attention and immediate action. The instruments for resolution of the immediate problem can be developed best at the national level with strong input from the subnational regions.

Long term planning, however, which would attempt to integrate health manpower planning with health services planning must begin at the national level but clearly needs transnational coordination. Implementation, again, requires powerful inputs from the infranational regions.

Recommendation Number 1

A message should be sent to each national government of the Community to urge each to establish a permanent working body having the following functions:

A) introduce measures to alleviate as quickly as possible the problems associated with physician unemployment;

B) establish continuing mechanisms for collecting and analysing information relevant to an integrated planning program for health services and health man power development in their country;

C) establish within each country a regional network or organization to make certain that each region of the country becomes intimately involved in the planning and implementation processes;

D) the national and regional bodies will have as their long term function the development of national policy on health services and manpower which is consistent with and coordinated with that of other member nations of the European Economic Community.

Recommendation Number 2

A message should be sent to each national government of the Community and to the European Economic Community to urge the establishment of a permanent forum at the EEC level for intensive study and discussion of health manpower, health education, and health services planning and policy. Close liaison with the World Health Organization should be sought. The proposed EEC Body* should collect and analyse relevant information, publish its conclusions on a regular basis, and serve a basic function of heightening EEC awareness of the necessity of transnational planning for health.

One aim of this body, urgently needed, is to develop trans-european guidelines to coordinate the health manpower legislation currently in process of being formulated by member nations of the EEC.

Close working linkages between the regional-national bodies in each country and the transnational body is required.

Ladies and gentlemen,

I have enjoyed and profited from the opportunity of participating in this conference.

* The body or forum referred to could be the Advisory Committee on Medical Training and the Committee of Senior Officials on Public Health of the EEC (75/364/EEC and 75/365/EEC, June 16, 1975) with expanded functions and membership.

Members of the Programma Committee

E.L. Vrijland, M.D.
Chairman of the Programme Committee
Neurologist, Senior Medical Officer of Health
Ministry of Health and Environmental Protection
Leidschendam, The Netherlands

Fr.C.A. Jaspers, M.D.
Secretary of the Programme Committee
Junior Hospital Doctor in Training for Internal Medicine
University Hospital, Department of Internal Medicine
Utrecht, The Netherlands

S.A. Duursma, M.D., Ph.D.
Professor of Internal Medicine
University Hospital, Department of Internal Medicine
Utrecht, The Netherlands

J.B.M. Edelman Bos, Ph.D.
Professor of Organizational Strategy
Graduate School of Management
Delft, The Netherlands
Director of the Management
Consultants Bosboom & Hegener NV
Amsterdam, The Netherlands

J.M. Greep, M.D., Ph.D.
Professor of Surgery
St Annadal University Hospital
Department of General Surgery
Dean of the Faculty of Medicine of the University Limburg
Maastricht,The Netherlands

A. Milton, M.D.
Pharmacologist
University of Uppsala
Department of Medical Pharmacology
Uppsala, Sweden

A.C. Nieuwenhuijzen Kruseman, M.D., Ph.D.
Registrar in Internal Medicine
University Hospital
Department of Endocrinology
Leyden, The Netherlands

A. Querido, M.D., Ph.D.
Professor of Internal Medicine
University Hospital
Department of Endocrinology
Leyden, The Netherlands

E. Reerink, M.D., Ph.D.
Director of the Central Institute on Medical Audit
Utrecht, The Netherlands

Members of the Organizing Committee

Fr.C.A. Jaspers, M.D.
Chairman of the Organizing Committee
Junior Hospital Doctor in Training for Internal Medicine
University Hospital, Department of Internal Medicine
Utrecht, The Netherlands

Ms E.B.J. de Groot, M.A. Law
Secretary of the Organizing Committee
Assistant of the Dean of the Faculty of Medicine
of the University Limburg
Maastricht, The Netherlands

D.B. van Egmond, M.D.
Treasurer of the Organizing Committee
Junior Hospital Doctor in Training for Surgery
University Hospital, Department of General Surgery
Leyden, The Netherlands

E.L. Vrijland, M.D.
Neurologist, Senior Medical Officer of Health
Ministry of Health and Environmental Protection
Leidschendam, The Netherlands

Contributors

M.E. Abrams, M.D., B.Sc., F.R.C.P.
Senior Principal Medical Officer
Department of Health and Social Security
Eileen House
80, Newington Canseway
London, United Kingdom

W. Albeda, Ph.D.
Social Economist, Former Minister of Social Affairs
Member of the Senate of The Netherlands
35, Jan van Ghestellaan
Rotterdam, The Netherlands

R. Brearley, M.S., F.R.C.S.
Member of the Standing Committee of Doctors of the EEC
Member of the Advisory Committee on Medical Training of the EEC
33, Queens Drive
Mossley Hill
Liverpool, United Kingdom

E. Duchene, M.D.
Conseiller National de l'Ordre National des Médécins
63, Boulevard de Latour-Maubourg
Paris, France

B. Eklundh, Ph.D.
Consultant in Health Manpower Planning and Management
at the Regional Office for Europe of the World Health Organization
8, Scherfigsvej
Copenhagen, Denmark

J.R. Evans, M.D., Ph.D.
Director of the Population, Health and Nutrition
Department of the World Bank
1818, H. Street, N.W.
Washington D.C., United States of America

P.A. Farrelly, M.D., Ph.D.
President of the Standing Committee of Doctors of the EEC
President of the Advisory Committee on Medical Training of the EEC
10, Fitzwilliam Place
Dublin, Ireland

I. Forgács, M.D., Ph.D.
Professor of Medicine
Director of the Research Unit for Education of the Semmelweis University of Medicine
Deputy Director-General of the Ministry of Health of Hungary
4, Nagyvárad ter
Budapest, Hungary

T. Fülöp, M.D., Ph.D.
Director of the Division of Health Manpower Development of the World Health Organization
Geneva, Switzerland

Mrs M.H.M.F. Gardeniers
Minister of Health and Environmental Protection of The Netherlands
12, Dr Reijersstraat
Leidschendam, The Netherlands

J.M. Greep, M.D., Ph.D.
Professor of Surgery
Head of the Department of General Surgery of the St Annadal (University) Hospital
Dean of the Faculty of Medicine of the University Limburg
P.O. Box 616
Maastricht, The Netherlands

R.B. Holmes, M.D.
Chairman of the Ontario Council of Health
Ministry of Health of Ontario
700, Bay Street
Toronto, Ontario, Canada

Fr.C.A. Jaspers, M.D.
Junior Hospital Doctor in Training for Internal Medicine
University Hospital Utrecht
Member of the Dutch Delegation in the Permanent Working Group of European Junior Hospital Doctors and the Standing Committee of Doctors of the EEC
Former President of the Dutch Association of Junior Hospital Doctors
698, Livingstonelaan
Utrecht, The Netherlands

R.M. Lapré, Ph.D.
Economist
Professor in Health Sciences
Secretary of the National Board of Health
Faculty of Medicine, Erasmus University
50, Dr Molewaterplein
Rotterdam, The Netherlands

A. Milton, M.D.
Pharmacologist, Department of Medical Pharmacology
University of Uppsala
Former President of the Swedish Association of Junior Hospital Doctors
Member of the Swedish Delegation in the Permanent Working Group of European Junior Hospital Doctors
59, Noreens Väg
Uppsala, Sweden

Dev.K. Ray, M.D., Ph.D.
Chief Scientist Health Manpower Planning of the Division of Health Manpower Development of the World Health Organization
Geneva, Switzerland

Mrs M. Schleicher, M.A. Law
Ministerialrätin im Bundesministerium für Jugend, Familie und Gesundheit
105-107, Kennedy Allee
Bonn, Federal Republic of Germany

A. Seiler,M.D.
Nefrologist, Coordinating Secretary of the Permanent Working Group of European Junior Hospital Doctors
5, Neuengasse
Berne, Switzerland

A.R. Tarlov, M.D., Ph.D.
Professor of Medicine
Head of the Section of General Internal Medicine
University of Chicago
Chairman of the Graduate Medical Educational National Advisory Committee (GMENAC) of the U.S.A.
950, East 59th Street
Chicago, Illinois, United States of America

E.L. Vrijland, M.D.
Neurologist, Senior Medical Officer of Health
Former President of the Dutch Association of Junior Hospital Doctors
Former Member of the Dutch Delegation in the Permanent Working Group of European Junior Hospital Doctors
20, Hugo de Grootstraat
Leyden, The Netherlands

G.A. Wagner, M.A. Law
Chairman of the Supervisory Board of the Royal Dutch Petroleum Company
30, Carel van Bijlandtlaan
The Hague, The Netherlands

Sponsors

This symposium and the publication of its proceedings were made possible by the support of the:

- Association des Médecins-Dentistes du Grand-Duché de Luxembourg, Luxemburg
- Bonifex, Projectontwikkeling en Promotie NV, The Netherlands
- Byk Nederland BV Farmaca, The Netherlands
- Capaciteitsgroep Algemene Heelkunde, Faculteit der Geneeskunde, Rijksuniversiteit Limburg, The Netherlands
- Crediet- en Effectenbank NV, The Netherlands
- Koninklijke Luchtvaart Maatschappij NV (KLM), The Netherlands
- Koninklijke Nederlandsche Maatschappij tot bevordering der Geneeskunst (KNMG), The Netherlands
- Landelijke vereniging van Artsen in Dienstverband (LAD), The Netherlands
- Landelijke Vereniging van Assistent-Geneeskundigen (LVAG), The Netherlands
- Landelijke Specialisten Vereniging (LSV), The Netherlands
- Ministerie van Onderwijs en Wetenschappen, The Netherlands
- Ministerie van Sociale Zaken en Werkgelegenheid, The Netherlands
- Ministerie van Volksgezondheid en Milieuhygiëne, The Netherlands
- Nederlandse Associatie van de Farmaceutische Industrie (NEFARMA), The Netherlands
- NV Levensverzekering Maatschappij 'Utrecht' (AMEV-groep), The Netherlands
- NV Verzekering Maatschappij 'Holland' (AMEV-groep), The Netherlands
- Shell Nederland BV, The Netherlands
- Stichting Overleg Limburgse Ziekenfondsen, The Netherlands
- Sveriges Yngre Läkares Förening (SYLF), Sweden

GPSR Compliance
The European Union's (EU) General Product Safety Regulation (GPSR) is a set of rules that requires consumer products to be safe and our obligations to ensure this.

If you have any concerns about our products, you can contact us on

ProductSafety@springernature.com

In case Publisher is established outside the EU, the EU authorized representative is:

Springer Nature Customer Service Center GmbH
Europaplatz 3
69115 Heidelberg, Germany

www.ingramcontent.com/pod-product-compliance
Ingram Content Group UK Ltd.
Pitfield, Milton Keynes, MK11 3LW, UK
UKHW022108180926
475695UK00001B/52
* 9 7 8 9 4 0 0 9 6 6 9 5 6 *